Ear, Nose and
Throat Nursing

Current Nursing Practice Titles

Ear, Nose and Throat Nursing

Agnes E. Stalker, BA, DipNEd, RGN, RNT, RCNT, ONC

Senior Tutor, Post Basic Courses, Western
College of Nursing and Midwifery, Glasgow;
External Examiner of ENT course approved by
the National Board for Nursing, Midwifery
and Health Visiting for Scotland

Sixth edition

Baillière Tindall **London Philadelphia Toronto
Mexico City Rio de Janeiro Sydney Tokyo Hong Kong**

Baillière Tindall   1 St Anne's Road
W. B. Saunders   Eastbourne, East Sussex BN21 3UN, England

West Washington Square
Philadelphia, PA 19105, USA

1 Goldthorne Avenue
Toronto, Ontario M8Z 5T9, Canada

Apartado 26370—Cedro 512
Mexico 4, DF Mexico

Rua Evaristo da Veiga 55, 20° andar
Rio de Janeiro—RJ, Brazil

ABP Australia Ltd, 44 Waterloo Road
North Ryde, NSW 2113, Australia

Ichibancho Central Building, 22–1 Ichibancho
Chiyoda-ku, Tokyo 102, Japan

10/FL, Inter-Continental Plaza, 94 Granville Road
Tsim Sha Tsui East, Kowloon, Hong Kong

© 1984 Baillière Tindall. All rights reserved. No part of this publication may be reproduced,
stored in a retrieval system or transmitted, in any form or by any means, electronic, mechanical,
photocopying or otherwise, without the prior permission of Baillière Tindall, 1 St Anne's Road,
Eastbourne, East Sussex BN21 3UN, England

First published in Nurses' Aids Series 1953
5th edition 1972
6th edition 1984
Spanish edition of 4th edition (CECSA, Mexico), 1970
Portuguese edition of 5th edition (Publicacoes Europa-America, Mira-Sintra), 1983

Typeset by Eta Services (Typesetters) Ltd., Beccles, Suffolk
Printed and bound in Great Britain by
Richard Clay (The Chaucer Press) Ltd
Bungay, Suffolk

British Library Cataloguing in Publication Data

Stalker, Agnes E.
  Ear, nose and throat nursing.—6th ed.
  —(Current nursing practice)
  1. Otolaryngology   2. Otolaryngological nursing
  I. Title   II. Marshall, Suzanna
  617'.51'0024613   RF46

ISBN 0–7020–1051–0

Contents

Preface

The main aim of this book is to present the subject of Ear, Nose and Throat Nursing in a coherent manner, so that the nurse, while undertaking her basic training, may learn what is normal, and so recognize the abnormal. It is also intended as a handbook for the nurse on an advance course in the UK, and for nursing colleagues in the rest of Europe and the Third World.

I have concentrated on bringing this new edition up to date, but have kept in mind the value placed on previous editions by nursing colleagues from countries which are not so advanced medically or technically.

Those wishing to go more deeply into this specialized field of Ear, Nose and Throat nursing should make reference to any of the excellent texts available, some of which are listed at the end of this edition.

Nan Stalker

Acknowledgement

Many of the line drawings in Appendix B, Glossary of Instruments, are taken from Macarthys' catalogue of Instruments for Ear, Nose and Throat Surgery (no. 7).

I Introduction

1 Preventative measures in ear, nose and throat care

Patients suffering from diseases of the ear, nose and throat are best nursed in a special section of a general hospital. The department, commonly spoken of as 'Ear, Nose and Throat', is often labelled 'Department of Otolaryngology' or given an even more elaborate title, and as some of the work is carried out in semi-darkness, nurses are apt to look upon work in such a department as shrouded in mystery. The principles of nursing the patient are, however, exactly the same as in other branches of medicine and surgery. A knowledge of the positions and interrelations of the structures involved will considerably help the nurse to 'unravel the mystery'. Detailed anatomy will be given in the special sections of this book. This chapter will introduce the nurse to the body's natural measures to prevent ear, nose and throat problems.

Mucous membrane: a protective mechanism

The continuous layer of mucous membrane which lines the ear, nose and throat is vitally important to the health of the individual. It lines the nasal cavities, with the exception of the vestibules and is firmly blended with the periosteum and perichondrium of their walls. It lines the lacrimal duct and is continuous with the conjunctiva. It extends throughout the pharynx, to the middle ear via the pharyngotympanic (*Eustachian*) tube, throughout the air sinuses, the larynx and lower air passages, and also, although we are not concerned with this part of the body at the moment, it lines the alimentary canal. (See Fig. 1.1.)

Over the conchae and septum of the nose, the mucous membrane is very thick and vascular, but it is thin on the floor of the nose, in the meatuses and in the air sinuses. In the pharynx and larynx it is more loosely attached, with a considerable amount of submucous tissue, but below the level of the vocal cords it is once more closely adherent to the underlying structures. Owing to the thickness of the

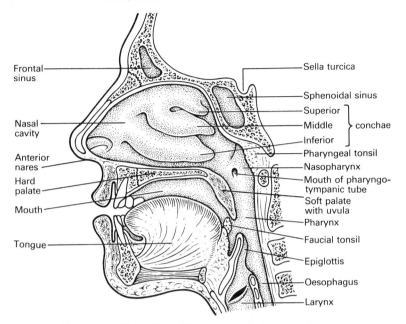

Fig. 1.1. *Sagittal section of the nose, mouth, pharynx and larynx.*

mucous membrane, the nasal cavities are narrower and the conchae more prominent than they appear in the skeleton. In inflammatory conditions, the membrane is liable to be very swollen from effusion. With a cold in the nose this is commonly sufficient to block the nasal passages completely. A much more dangerous state can arise with 'oedema of the glottis'; the larynx may be occluded and asphyxia result. Oedema of the glottis (especially in the subglottic space and loose tissue around the arytenoids) occurs also with non-inflammatory affections such as giant urticaria and serum sickness.

The mucous membrane is well supplied with blood vessels and in most parts contains many *mucous glands*, some 'goblet cell' in type and some tubulo-alveolar, which open on its surface.

The mucus secreted by these glands keeps the membrane moist. The epithelium forming the surface layer of cells in the respiratory tract is mainly columnar and ciliated. These *cilia* are microscopic projections from the free surface of the epithelial cell, and, in health, are in constant motion. They act in sections, moving forward quickly and back slowly, from eight to twelve times per second. With the strong forward movement, the cilia brush along the mucus, with which are entangled dust and bacteria. In the nose, the mucus is propelled toward the pharynx; in the bronchial tree, the direction is toward the glottis. The hairs in the nostrils filter the larger particles of foreign matter from the inspired air, and the cilia complete this important cleansing function. The cilia may continue to beat strongly in the presence of infection and pus, and are commonly regenerated with the epithelium following damage to the membrane. They are slowed down with cooling and over-heating but recover when the normal temperature returns. However, drying and smoking are fatal to them. In chronic inflammation, such as that of the paranasal sinuses, the epithelium becomes so damaged that the cilia disappear. This interferes with the normal self-cleansing function, and operations have often to be performed to allow the pus which accumulates to escape.

Breathing habits

Upon the integrity of the mucous membrane depends a great deal of man's resistance to infection, and to preserve it is the aim of preventive measures in ear, nose and throat work. A most important factor in health is correct breathing. When 'out of breath' after strenuous exercise one may take in supplementary air through the mouth, but in quiet breathing the tidal air should pass freely in and out of the nose. It is sometimes necessary to close the mouth of a sleeping infant so that it shall learn to breathe correctly. Mouth breathing begins a vicious circle. Air that is inspired through the nose is drawn through the hairs inside the vestibule. It is then warmed and moistened as it passes over the mucous surfaces. Air inhaled through the mouth lacks this filtration, warmth and moisture, and the lining of the pharynx on which the cold air strikes deteriorates in the attempt to react to such unfavourable conditions. A degree of inflammation is set up, causing enlargement of the adenoids. This in turn obstructs the nasal passages, so that breathing through them is impossible and the child perforce becomes an habitual mouth breather.

The use of handkerchiefs

As early in life as possible, a child should be taught to use a handkerchief properly. Very often the sole instruction given is by a slightly older brother or sister, who holds the handkerchiefs, nips the infant's nose and says firmly 'Now, blow!'. This most admirable effort at education needs to be supplemented by a parent or nurse. The correct method of blowing the nose is to compress each nostril alternately and blow down the other. To blow forcibly down both at once while the nostrils are closed is liable to send infectious material into the middle ear via the pharyngotympanic tube.

Each child should be provided with his own handkerchief and supervised to ensure that it is not used as a shoe polisher, duster or paint rag! Should there be much nasal discharge, as in a head cold, paper handkerchiefs should be used by old as well as young, care being taken to ensure that the soiled ones are disposed of efficiently.

Constant use of a handkerchief that is harsh either by reason of its texture or because of dried nasal discharge will cause soreness of the upper lip or painful fissures around the vestibule. When linen or cotton handkerchiefs are used during respiratory infection, they should be disinfected before being washed and boiled. Dettol is a satisfactory disinfectant if the handkerchiefs are immersed in it for eight hours.

Respiratory infection

Most respiratory and many other diseases begin with the *common cold*, spread by droplet infection — that is, micro-organisms from one person's nose and throat projected in a fine spray of saliva to the mucous membrane of a second person. There, should the second person be susceptible, they will penetrate and multiply. The common cold is the greatest cause that exists of loss of time from occupation and therefore much research has been devoted to discovering its cause and toward preventing its spread.

Since the use of the electron microscope, it has been found that several strains of virus may cause the common cold. Experiments upon healthy individuals living in strict isolation have proved that these viruses are responsible for the early symptoms — that is, the nasal irritation, the dry sensation (generally in the nasopharynx), the sneezing, followed in a few hours by profuse discharge of watery mucus, and general malaise. After a simple virus infection there is a gradual return to normal in three to seven days. In ordinary life the individual is exposed to other pathogenic bacteria, such as *Neisseria catarrhalis*, streptococcus, staphylococcus, pneumococcus and *Haemophilus influenzae*. It is the increase of these organisms that appears to be responsible for the more advanced symptoms of a cold — the purulent nasal discharge, the sore throat and the sinusitis.

There are several known predisposing factors. In over-heated rooms, the air tends to dry the film of mucus covering the nasal and oral cavities. The cilia, which move the mucus, and with it, the dust and germs, then becomes less active. The dried mucus forms crusts inside the nostrils, and there, especially if the nose is picked with the finger-nail, is a potential site for the entrance of pathogenic bacteria. Sometimes anatomical abnormalities, such as deviation of the septum, so alter air currents inside the nose that they impinge on one spot in the posterior nares and so cause drying.

Defence against infection

Experiments at the Common Cold Research Unit have disproved many long-standing preconceptions as to the causes of colds, such as exposure to cold or long standing in wet garments. However, clothing appears to be a factor in relation to respiratory infections, especially in children. Underclothing should be light in weight and loosely woven to enmesh air which is a poor conductor of heat. As few garments should be worn as are consistent with comfort. In cold weather warm coats and strong shoes should be provided for outdoor wear, and children must not be expected to be too 'hardy'. A quick reaction of the skin to changes in temperature is something to be encouraged, but it must not be presumed to be automatic in all individuals or to occur too early in life.

The general resistance to infection also depends on an *adequate, well-balanced diet*. Regular, wholesome meals are essential to health, and extra vitamins, especially A, C and D, are protective against respiratory infections. Ascorbic acid, cod-liver oil and malt, or similar preparations containing vitamins, can be taken over the winter months, but only as a supplement to the normal diet. The habit of omitting breakfast and having a 'snack lunch' predisposes to infections of the respiratory tract. It leads to fatigue — another factor that lowers resistance.

Adequate hours of sleep in a ventilated room, with warm but not heavy bedclothes, are essential to health. It is important to avoid overcrowding and to maintain good ventilation in all situations of work, leisure, sleep and meals. During outbreaks of respiratory infectious diseases, the avoidance of crowded public places, such as cinemas and large department stores should be strongly recommended.

Attempts have been made, with some success, to create an immunity to colds by the injection of vaccines. For some specific diseases — diphtheria, whooping cough, poliomyelitis — vaccines are widely used, particularly in early life.

The spread of respiratory infection

During quiet breathing the range of droplet spread is usually 2–3 m, but droplets may be carried 18 m or more by currents of air. The spread is much increased by the sneezing and coughing, with which so many infectious diseases commence. It is during the onset of the disease, therefore, that persons are most highly infectious.

There are a variety of pathogenic organisms which tend to multiply in the mucous membrane of the nose and throat. Many individuals harbour organisms to which they themselves are immune, but which may produce clinical attacks in others. Such individuals are known as 'carriers'. Diseases commonly transmitted by carriers are the various manifestations of infection by the haemolytic streptococcus, diphtheria caused by the corynaebacterium diphtheriae, and cerebrospinal meningitis caused by the meningococcus. Recently the carriage of *Staphylococcus aureus* (often resistant to antibiotics) in the nostrils has assumed great importance in hospital and carriers are excluded from contact with wounds. It must be borne in mind that haemolytic streptococci are responsible for many diseases including scarlet fever, tonsillitis, cervical adenitis, sinusitis, otitis media, mastoiditis, skin sepsis, impetigo, wound suppuration, cellulitis, erysipelas, puerperal fever and septicaemia. All patients with such diseases should be nursed by isolation technique, preferably in a single room or in a cubicle. If possible, all nurses attending them should be immune.

2 Infection control in the Ear, Nose and Throat Unit

Layout of Unit

An ideal Ear, Nose and Throat Unit should be self-contained, consisting of an Out-Patients' Department, an operating theatre equipped with its own anaesthetic and instrument rooms, and wards for in-patients. There may be a separate dressing room and a postoperative intensive care unit. The spacing of the beds in the wards is an important consideration. The incidence of carriers is greatly increased by overcrowding, and cross-infection becomes inevitable in a ward where beds are too close together. The distance between the bed centres should be not less than 3.6 m or, if beds face each other, there should be 5.2 m between the two heads. Wards are best subdivided by glazed screens 2.35 m high, with a 15 cm clearance of the floor for ease of cleaning, into some single-bedded cubicles (particularly in the section for young children) and some four-bedded wards. This limits the spread of infection and ensures more privacy and quiet for the patients, who can at the same time be under observation by the nursing staff through the glass partitions. The wards should be light and airy, and the ventilation as free as possible. In some units, a Plenum ventilation system is installed, providing positive pressure in treatment rooms, negative in the sluice room. If the beds are placed parallel to the long axis of the ward, the patients do not directly face the light. Often balconies or verandas are provided, and patients should be encouraged to use these both winter and summer. Even if balconies are not available, almost open-air conditions can be achieved in the ward if one or more walls are largely windows.

Cross-infection and its prevention

Ward dust contains millions of bacteria. These are mostly harmless, but pathogenic organisms are usually present. In the Ear, Nose and Throat ward of one hospital the floor sweepings were estimated to contain 100 000 000 haemolytic streptococci. Staphylococci, diphtheria bacilli, pneumococci and tubercle bacilli have also been found. The bacteria emanate from bedclothes, personal clothes and dried droplets. Blankets of patients with upper respiratory infections harbour a great many germs which are scattered into the air at every bedmaking or movement of the blankets or duvet. Dust that is raised settles again to contaminate furniture, bedclothes, patient's clothing, or be inhaled by persons in the ward.

Should pathogenic organisms be present in sufficient quantities, and should they fall on susceptible tissues, infection will thus be spread.

Ward hygiene

In order to reduce dust-borne infection, ward cleaning should be done by vacuum and damp dusting. No dry dusting should be allowed.

Wool blankets are now largely replaced by cotton or cellular weave, and many hospitals now use duvets. Blankets are easily washed, and duvets can be dry-cleaned.

Soiled linen should be put into bags at the bedside; the bags then being sealed and taken to the laundry.

Nursing principles

The nursing staff must apply aseptic principles to their work at all times.

When working with a patient, the nurse should wash and dry her hands before and after each procedure. Linen roller towels can harbour infection, and disposable paper towels should be used if available.

Efficient face masks should be worn by the staff when carrying out aseptic procedures. The mask should cover nose, mouth and chin. Face masks are usually disposable and should be discarded after use; they should never be kept in the nurse's pocket.

Should an outbreak of an infectious disease occur in a ward, all patients showing signs of the infection should be barrier nursed or sent to an isolation unit. Antiserum is given to those postoperative patients who have not had the infection. All those who are particularly susceptible to the infection should be kept under close observation.

During the incubation period of the disease, all patients should be kept in bed and examined for early signs and symptoms. The admission of new patients should cease until there is no danger of further spread of the infection. For example, if diphtheria occurs, no new patients should be admitted; if whooping cough occurs, no new patients under three years of age should be admitted. The admission of children for tonsillectomy should also be suspended when severe epidemics, e.g. of poliomyelitis, measles or scarlet fever, are prevalent in the neighbourhood. The operation should not be performed on children who have not been immunized against poliomyelitis.

The noses, throats, wounds or discharges should be examined bacteriologically, and the patients should not be regarded as free from infection until at least two successive negative swabs, at an interval of not less than three days, have been obtained. All members of the ward staff who show any sign or symptom of infection by haemolytic streptococci — whether it is sore throat, severe cold, skin sepsis (especially of fingers) or other manifestation — should be taken off duty until they have ceased to be carriers. However willing a nurse may be to sacrifice herself to her duty, she must remember that when she is not well she may be a serious danger to her patients, and should therefore not delay in reporting early signs of infection. This is particularly important in an Ear, Nose and Throat Unit, where many of the patients are children whose immunity is not fully developed. The majority of patients, moreover, are already suffering from an inflammation of the mucous membrane and are therefore susceptible to infections other than those causing the original disease. Should a chronic carrier of infection — that is, one who harbours the germ long after all signs of the disease have disappeared — be found among the staff, he or she must be excluded from the ward.

II The Ear

3 Anatomy of the ear

The ear is divided anatomically into three parts: *the outer ear*, consisting of the auricle or pinna and the external auditory meatus, which is a passage leading to the eardrum; *the middle ear*, which is a roughly spherical cavity about the size of a large pea, situated within the temporal bone, internal to the eardrum and containing the three auditory ossicles; and *the inner ear*, which is situated deep within the temporal bone and is connected via the internal auditory meatus to the central nervous system by the auditory (8th cranial) nerve, which has two distinct parts, the cochlear, concerned with hearing, and the vestibular, concerned with the sense of balance. (See Fig. 3.1.)

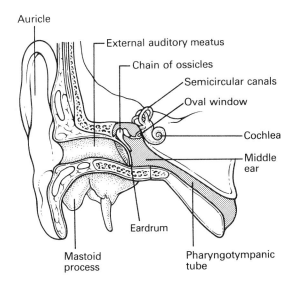

Auricle
External auditory meatus
Chain of ossicles
Semicircular canals
Oval window
Cochlea
Middle ear
Eardrum
Mastoid process
Pharyngotympanic tube

Fig. 3.1. *View of the right ear with the outer and middle ear seen in section during swallowing. (Except when swallowing, the mouth of the pharyngotympanic tube is closed.)*

THE OUTER EAR

The auricle

Except in the lobe, the auricle (Fig. 3.2) is made up of an irregular plate of elastic cartilage covered by skin. It is attached to the temporal bone by ligaments and is continuous with the cartilage of the auditory meatus. There are some muscular attachments, but very little movement of the outer ear occurs in man; it is purely

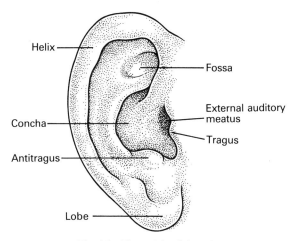

Fig. 3.2. *The auricle of the ear.*

ornamental. In other animals, such as the dog, the auricle is moved in order to catch sound waves. On the anterior surface of the auricle the skin adheres closely to the cartilage, which accounts for the frequent occurrence of haematoma following injury of this surface, but on the posterior surface it is looser. The free lobe of the ear is a particular characteristic of man.

The auricle is supplied with blood from the posterior auricular artery behind and the superficial temporal artery in front. The superficial position of the vessels in the thin skin and the lack of subcutaneous tissue and fat make the auricle particularly susceptible to frostbite.

The sensory nerves supplying the auricle are branches from the mandibular division of the trigeminal nerve, the lesser occipital and great auricular nerves from the cervical plexus, and the auricular branch of the vagus nerve. The muscles of the auricle are supplied by the facial nerve.

The external auditory meatus

The external auditory meatus begins as a funnel-shaped opening in the auricle and leads inwards to the temporal bone, where it is closed by the tympanic (or drum-like) membrane. The latter is placed obliquely so that the canal of an adult is about 26 mm long on the superoposterior wall and 32 mm long on the anteroinferior wall. Wax frequently collects in the lower corner so formed. The meatus is in the shape of an elongated and twisted S, the direction being first upward, inward and forward. It soon bends inward and backward, then downward, inward and backward. To straighten and make the eardrum visible, it is necessary to pull the auricle upward and backward. The outer third, or rather more, of the auditory canal is cartilaginous; the remainder lies in the temporal bone. The entire canal is linked by skin. There are two constrictions in the canal, one near the medial end of the cartilaginous portion, the other in the osseous portion. Near the auricle, the skin lining the canal is set with hairs, while within, in the subcutaneous tissue of the cartilaginous portion, are numerous ceruminous glands which secrete wax. The hairs help to prevent the entrance of insects, and by means of the wax insects and bacteria are entangled. Absence of wax occurs in disease. An accumulation of wax may block the passage and cause deafness. In the bony portion of the external auditory meatus the skin is thin, devoid of hairs and contains very few wax glands. The shortness of the meatus in children, before the skull bones have fully ossified, must be remembered when examining with an aural speculum, lest the eardrum be damaged.

THE MIDDLE EAR

The middle ear or tympanic cavity is an air-containing cavity, hollowed out in the substance of the temporal bone and is separated from the outer ear by the tympanic membrane or eardrum.

The tympanic membrane

The tympanic membrane is an exceedingly thin, pearly grey,

semitransparent, almost circular membrane, which has a vertical
diameter of about 10 mm and a horizontal diameter of about
7.5 mm. Its circumference is slightly thickened and forms a fibro-
cartilaginous ring by which it is attached to the medial end of the
external auditory meatus. The inner surface of the membrane is
convex, and to the point of greatest convexity is attached the tip of
the malleus, the first of the chain of ossicles which crosses the middle
ear (see Fig. 3.3). Below this point, on examining the ear from the

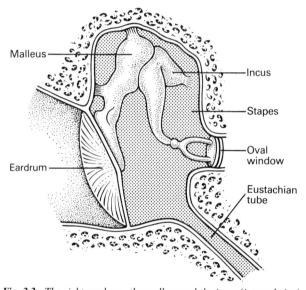

Fig. 3.3. *The right eardrum, the malleus and the incus (internal view).*

meatus inwards by reflected light, a brightly illuminated 'cone of
light' can be seen over the anteroinferior quadrant of the membrane.
Here the eardrum presents a plane surface to the light rays, with no
structure to obscure its translucency. There is a small, somewhat
triangular, loose area (Shrapnell's membrane) in the upper part of
the eardrum but the main part of the drum is tightly stretched.
Although the drum is so thin, it consists of four layers:

1. The outer layer of stratified epithelium, derived from the skin
   lining the external auditory meatus.
2. A layer of radiating white connective tissue fibres.

3. A layer of circular fibres, thicker around the circumference.

4. The mucous membrane lining the middle ear.

In the flaccid part of the eardrum the fibrous tissue is absent, and this is therefore the weakest part of the eardum.

The roof of the middle ear is formed by a thin plate of bone — part of the anterior surface of the petrous portion of the temporal bone — which separates it from the cranial cavity. On the *inner wall* there are two small openings, the oval window (fenestra ovalis) and the round window (fenestra rotunda). Both of these are closed by membranes. They lead to the internal ear — the oval window to the vestibule and the round window to the cochlea.

From the anterior wall, near the floor of the middle ear, passing inwards and forwards, is the pharyngotympanic tube, long known as the Eustachian tube. This tube is about 40 mm long and leads into the nasopharynx. Through it, air enters the middle ear. The posterior third of the tube is surrounded by the temporal bone, and the anterior two-thirds are partly cartilaginous and partly fibrous. The tube is closed except in the action of swallowing. Then, the flaccid walls of the tube are pulled apart by the action of one of the swallowing muscles. A cold in the nose sometimes spreads up the pharyngotympanic tube and the swollen mucous membrane blocks the tube. As a result the air in the middle ear cannot be renewed; it becomes absorbed by the blood in the capillaries, and the pressure of the air outside the tympanic membrane is no longer counterbalanced by the air within. The membrane is then pulled in tightly and cannot vibrate. This causes the deafness that is so common in people with heavy colds. In children the pharyngotympanic tube is more horizontal than in adults and therefore infection can pass from the nose to the middle ear more easily.

Mastoid air cells

The middle ear cavity also opens into an air space in the mastoid process, known as the mastoid antrum, which in turn opens into other air cells. These air spaces develop in growing bone in the same way as the paranasal sinuses and are similarly lined with mucous membrane. The mastoid process is recognizable as a bony prominence towards the end of the second year. In an adult, whose mastoid air cells are completely developed, the prominence is large and rounded. Frequently, however, development is retarded, the air cells being small or absent and the process small. The bony roof of the mastoid antrum is extremely thin, especially in a child, and infection in the middle ear and mastoid antrum may spread to the dura mater of the cranial fossa.

Auditory ossicles

Across the cavity of the middle ear are strung three exquisitely small bones called the auditory ossicles. These are: the malleus or hammer, the incus or anvil, and the stapes or stirrup, being named after objects they resemble. They are attached to each other by ligaments. The rounded head of the malleus is jointed to a hollow in the incus, and the long arm of the incus is similarly jointed to the stapes. The long handle of the malleus is attached to the eardrum, and the plate of the stapes is fixed to the membrane which closes the oval window. The line of attachment of the malleus is visible on the eardrum when examined through the external meatus. All three ossicles are covered by thin mucous membrane continuous with that lining the walls of the middle ear. There is a recess in the middle ear, lying above and behind the head of the malleus and the body of the incus, called the *attic* or *epitympanic recess*. This leads into the mastoid antrum and is important in cases of infection of the middle ear.

Sound waves, which cause the eardrum to vibrate, are generally thought to be amplified by the chain of ossicles and transmitted to the oval window. From here they travel through the inner ear and return to the round window. The physiology of hearing will be further described in the next chapter.

THE INNER EAR

The inner ear, or labyrinth, comprises a series of cavities and canals in the petrous portion of the temporal bone. The bony canals and spaces are called the *bony labyrinth* (Fig. 3.4). They are lined with periosteum and enclose the *membranous labyrinth*. The bony labyrinth is formed of three layers: an outer periosteal layer, a middle layer derived from the cartilage surrounding the embryonic membranous labyrinth, and an inner layer of endosteum. The inner layer has no blood vessels and is of ivory-like hardness. The adjacent side of the middle layer is also dense, but the external layer next to the periosteum is of looser texture. In the disease called otosclerosis, the changes in bone occur in this layer.

The different parts of the bony labyrinth are: the vestibule, the three semicircular canals, and the cochlea.

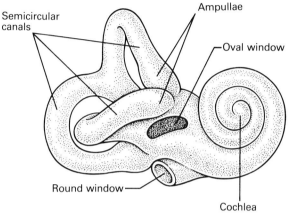

Fig. 3.4. *The bony labyrinth.*

The vestibule

The vestibule lies medially to the middle ear, its lateral wall being perforated by the oval and round windows. It is a small, irregular cavity, and the cochlea leads into it from the front and the semicircular canals from behind.

The semicircular canals

The three semicircular canals are very small hoops of bone, each forming about two-thirds of a circle and having a diameter of one millimetre except at one end where it dilates into an 'ampulla'. The canals are set at right angles to each other, in different planes. Their non-ampullated ends join to make a common entrance in the medial wall of the vestibule. The ampullae of the superior and lateral canals have their openings into the vestibule above the oval windows, whilst the posterior ampulla opens into it below the oval window.

The bony cochlea

The bony cochlea (Fig. 3.5) is a flattened cone, about 1 cm at its base. It is formed of a central column, the modiolus, around which a hollow spiral tube makes two and a half turns, like a snail shell. A delicate spiral shelf of bone projects from the modiolus into the canal and winds upwards to the apex. The shelf reaches about half-way across the canal, and partially divides it into two. The division is

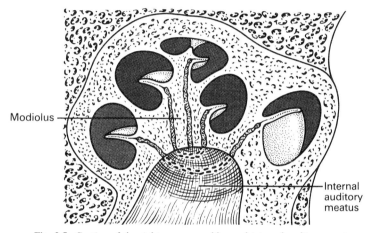

Fig. 3.5. *Section of the right osseous cochlea and internal auditory meatus.*

completed by a membrane called the basilar membrane, and the two canals communicate at the apex of the cochlea. In the modiolus are small openings through which pass branches of the cochlear nerve. The base of the cochlea has three openings: the opening into the vestibule, the round window, and a minute duct through which connection is made with the subarachnoid space.

The membranous labyrinth

The membranous labyrinth (Fig. 3.6) lies within the bony labyrinth, but is very much smaller. The space between it and the surrounding bone is occupied by *perilymph*, which is a fluid identical in composition and confluent with the cerebrospinal fluid. The membranous labyrinth contains fluid called *endolymph*, and in its walls the filaments of the auditory nerve are distributed. Inside the semicircular canals the membranous labyrinth closely follows the shape of the bone; in the vestibule it forms two sacs called the *utricle* and the *saccule*; in the cochlea it is arranged as a third spiral tube lying along the outer wall of the cochlea. (The double bony spiral of the cochlea contains perilymph, the membranous duct contains endolymph.)

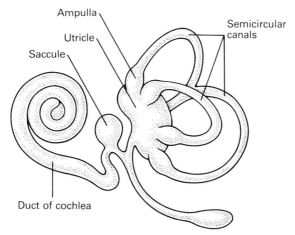

Fig. 3.6. *The membranous labyrinth (diagrammatic).*

The various parts of the membranous labyrinth form a closed system of channels which communicate with each other. In the case of the utricle, saccule and semicircular canals, the inner surface of the membranous labyrinth shows patches of neuroepithelial tissue — one in the utricle, one in the saccule and one in each ampulla. These patches consist of supporting cells and sensory cells with hair-like processes which project into the endolymph. Around these hair cells terminate the branches (peripheral processes) of the vestibular nerve — the central processes of this nerve mostly end in the medulla oblongata (vestibular nuclei) and in the cerebellum. Here secondary connections are made which govern the equilibrium of the body.

Within the cochlea lies the *organ of Corti*, the receiving apparatus for hearing. It is formed of highly specialized epithelial cells, making a tunnel of tiny arched rods, resting on the basilar membrane (see

Fig. 3.7). On either side of the tunnel are the sensory cells with hair-like processes. It has been estimated that there are nearly 10 000 of these rods, and twice that number of hair cells, within the spiral membranous labyrinth of the cochlea. The cochlear nerve fibres which terminate round the hair cells pass into the medulla oblongata and thence to the principal auditory centres in the cerebrum. The

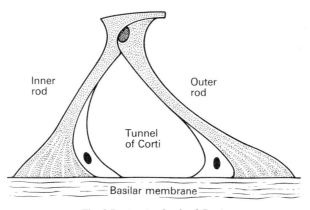

Fig. 3.7. *A pair of rods of Corti.*

cochlear and the vestibular nerves join before leaving the inner ear to form the auditory (eighth cranial) nerve. Although the cochlear nerve is that of hearing and the vestibular nerve that of balance, the two have some connections, and both can influence motor cells in the spinal cord.

The facial nerve in relation to the ear

The facial nerve, in part of its course, lies in so intimate a relation to the ear, that it is often involved in diseases of and operations upon the latter.

The seventh cranial (facial) and the eighth cranial (auditory) nerves emerge side by side from the brain at the lower border of the pons, and together enter the internal auditory meatus. At the bottom of the meatus, the facial nerve enters the facial canal, a bony groove in the temporal bone. This groove is first directed laterally between the vestibule and the cochlea of the ear, then it passes into the aditus, downwards in the posterior wall of the middle ear and so into the mastoid process.

Finally the facial nerve emerges through the stylomastoid foramen, and supplies the muscles of the face. It is therefore below and in front of the inner part of the mastoid antrum (see Fig. 3.8). Facial paralysis may result from caries of the bony wall of the middle ear.

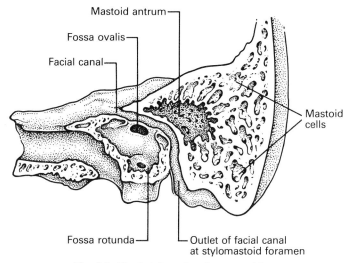

Fig. 3.8. *The facial canal in the temporal bone.*

In operative treatment, great care is necessary to avoid damaging the nerve.

In an infant, the mastoid process has not developed, so that the mastoid antrum lies above rather than behind the middle ear and the facial nerve emerges from the stylomastoid foramen beneath the skin, unprotected by the mastoid process. An incautious incision down to the bone may then cut the nerve.

A short distance before the facial nerve leaves the bone, a branch is given off to the middle ear, to a small muscle inserted into the stapes. This muscle is caused to contract reflexly in response to very loud sounds and so is able to some extent to protect the organ of Corti from noise injury.

4 Physiology of the ear and deafness

The functions of the ear are hearing and balance. Either or both of these are disturbed in diseases of the ear, and in order to understand them, the previous chapter should be studied. The physiology of the ear is briefly considered here.

THE PHYSIOLOGY OF HEARING

As with the other senses, hearing depends on four principal factors. There must be a stimulus, a receptor organ and a nerve pathway leading from the organ to the brain. In the temporal lobe of the brain there is an auditory area which receives the sensation of hearing and round it is an area which interprets what is heard.

In the sensory organ are the end-organs of the nerve fibres which, carrying the impulses along, form the nerves. The ear is the receptor organ of sound and in its innermost part, the inner ear, is the organ of Corti. This is composed of little hair-like structures, the end-organs of the sensory fibres, which are supported by the basilar membrane, a continuation from the bony platform spiralling round the central modiolus of the cochlea. The fibres pass via the bony ledge and the modiolus to the base of the cochlea and emerge as the auditory part of the eighth cranial nerve through the internal auditory meatus.

The external auditory meatus and the middle ear are constructed to carry the sound waves to the inner ear. Sound waves are disturbances in the air produced by a sounding body, e.g. a plucked violin string, a banging door or the human voice, very like the ripples raised on the surface of a pond if a stone is dropped into it. The ripples or vibrations are counted in numbers per second (hertz, Hz) the greater the number the higher the pitch, and vice versa. It is essential for the good conduction of sound that atmospheric pressure is equal on either side of the tympanic membrane separating the outer ear from the middle ear. The air in the middle ear comes up the pharyngotympanic tube (Eustachian tube); hence a blocked pharyngotympanic tube can produce deafness.

The waves of sound striking the tympanic membrane cause it to vibrate, and this movement is transmitted across the middle ear, usually through the body of the malleus and the short arm of the incus to the stapes. The footplate of the stapes, pushing the oval window in and out, sets up a travelling wave in the perilymph and along the basilar membrane. The perilymph is separated from the endolymph only by the upper membrane of the scala media, the membrane of Reissner. The swell therefore sets up a motion in the endolymph which rocks the basilar membrane and pulls on the sensitive hair cells of the organ of Corti. The wave ends at the round window which gives to accommodate it. Sound may reach the cochlea by vibrations conducted through the bones of the head, but a much greater intensity is needed for bone conduction than for air conduction.

Sensations of sound are distinguished by their loudness, their pitch and their quality. Loudness depends on the amplitude of vibrations; pitch, as already explained, upon the number of vibrations in a given time; quality, upon the regularity of the vibrations. A noise is the result of irregular vibrations, and a musical note is produced when the vibrations are orderly. The organ of Corti is responsible for separating the mixed vibrations which fall on the ear and converting each set into the corresponding nerve impulses.

For sound waves to pass freely through the ear, several factors are essential:

1. The tympanic membrane must be able to vibrate.
2. The pressure in the middle ear must equal that of the atmosphere.
3. The ossicles must be able to move.
4. The oval window and the round window must both be able to yield to the waves passing through the perilymph in the labyrinth of the inner ear.

Tinnitus is the sensation of hearing in the absence of external sound. It varies in pitch and character and may become extremely distressing. The cause may be anywhere in the path of transmission. It may be a lesion of the cochlea or some part of the auditory nerve and the condition may occur in many ear diseases or arise from the over-use of drugs such as quinine and the sodium salicylates including aspirin.

NOISE

There is considerable variation in the way in which different people react to noise. A sound volume which is acceptable to one person can be totally unacceptable to another. The factors which influence response to noise are both numerous and varied. The extrovert type of person who likes excitement may well find that music played at full volume is not only acceptable, but also pleasurable, while someone of more introvert nature, who is quiet and more reserved, may find the same volume quite intolerable. Similarly, the same loud music which gives pleasure to a young person, may well be an annoying noise to somebody in an older age group. Susceptibility to noise can also be affected by its cause. A man repairing or altering his home may not notice the noise created by his activity, but his neighbour who is trying to rest will not agree that the sounds are of reasonable level.

The judgement of sound intensity is subjective, and consequently the effects of noise are diverse. It can produce fatigue, frustration, irritation or considerable emotional disturbance. In certain instances it can result in actual damage to the ear and hearing loss. Exposure to noise of high intensity for a short period can result in auditory fatigue, which causes temporary deafness lasting several hours. Alternatively, in rare instances, it can rupture the tympanic membrane. This type of damage usually heals rapidly or is surgically repaired. Prolonged exposure to intense noise can result in damage to the inner ear. Such exposure damages the hair cells of the organ of Corti within the cochlea. There is decreased ability to hear higher pitched tones. At first the individual in unaware of this loss, and with continued exposure, further damage occurs. There will be difficulty in hearing speech in the higher frequencies (i.e. the consonants) of normal conversation. In consequence, the person misinterprets words and is unable to understand conversation. Later in life deafness due to advancing years may well aggravate the disability. Hearing aids are of little help to a noise-deaf person because they only amplify the sound without clarifying reception. In order to communicate, it is advisable to face the affected person and speak to him slowly and clearly without raising the voice unduly.

Where a person is subjected to continuous noise precautionary measures should be taken. For example, in industry a variety of methods of noise reduction are employed on machinery, which may be enclosed or muffled with acoustic, absorbent material. Where noise is a definite occupational hazard, ear muffs or plugs are provided to give protection. Not only are the employees encouraged to wear these, but the reason for their provision is carefully explained.

THE PHYSIOLOGY OF BALANCE

The ear is the organ of balance as well as of hearing. The receptor organs in this case are the semicircular canals, the saccule and the utricle. They are continuous with the membranous part of the cochlea and also contain endolymph.

The vestibular portion of the eighth cranial nerve contains the nerve fibres running from the end-organs, which lie in the ampullae of the semicircular canals, and the maculae of the saccule and utricle (see Fig. 3.6, p. 23), to the cerebellum, which co-ordinates the muscle movements controlling posture and balance. Two types of sensation are involved. The maculae are stimulated by alterations in the *position* of the head and supply some of the information necessary for regulating the muscle tone on which posture depends.

The semicircular canals are concerned with *movements* of the head. They lie horizontally, vertically and obliquely, and the endolymph filling them follows the movements of the head. Attached to the hair cells lining the membrane and projecting into this fluid are small particles of calcium carbonate called *otoliths*. The nerve endings in the ampullae are sensitive to alterations in fluid pressure produced by circular and rotary movements. The resulting stimuli travel along the nerve fibres to the cerebellum. The cerebellar response involves the organizing of the showers of impulses passing out from the cerebral cortex to opposing groups of muscles, so that whatever their activity, balance is maintained.

Hence injury or disease involving the labyrinths of the inner ear, e.g. Ménière's disease, will affect the power of balance. The patient suffers from a sense of falling or rotation (vertigo) which he attempts to counteract by muscular movements and therefore he staggers. It may be noted that pirouetting, swinging, and the pitching and tossing of a ship on the sea produce similar effects.

Vertigo, strictly meaning the sense of rotation, suggests dysfunction of the labyrinth or of the brain stem, whereas dizziness — the sensation of unsteadiness — is usually due to some reduction of the blood supply to the brain, as in fainting.

DEAFNESS

As will be understood from the preceding considerations, there are two types of deafness:

1. Conductive deafness — arising from an obstruction to the passage of sound waves.
2. Nerve deafness, the cause of which may rest in the nerve endings in the cochlea, in the auditory nerve or in the auditory cortex.

Differentiation between the two types may be difficult to achieve. The surgeon uses a tuning fork test to discover whether air-conduction is greater than bone conduction (as it should be) or vice versa. When deafness is present and the middle ear is shown to be normal by this test, the nerve type of deafness exists. Other tests are used to decide which ear is the more affected.

Accurate estimation of hearing is made by means of an audiometer, which is an instrument by which graphs can be charted showing the degree and type of hearing loss. The record is useful for future comparison for deciding on treatment and also for the provision of a hearing aid to suit the individual patient. The use of the audiometer demands a sound-proof room. Each ear is tested separately and the test takes twenty minutes or longer. Sound is produced electrically and the patient indicates the quietest sound that he can perceive at a given pitch.

When a patient is unequally deaf in the two ears, it is necessary to distinguish the hearing in the ear being tested from sounds heard by the opposite ear. For this purpose, Barany's noise box is used. This contains a small hammer which can be set to vibrate against a diaphragm. An ear-piece from the box is put into the ear not being tested and the noise of the vibration will mask the sounds being used for the hearing test on the opposite ear.

Hearing aids

A great number of hearing aids have been designed. The main

hearing aids used today are electrical aids, (a) of the valve type, (b) using transistors. These can be delicately adjusted to amplify sounds in accordance with the record of hearing obtained by audiometry. The varieties of electrical aids differ in pattern and weight in order to suit the daily living needs of the users. Body-level aids tend to be bulky; ear level aids are less conspicuous. In general, transistor aids are less cumbersome, less conspicuous, and give less distortion in amplification; also the batteries last longer.

Patients with hearing difficulties should never purchase a hearing aid without consulting an otologist.

5 Disorders of the outer ear

Otitis externa

Various skin diseases affect the outer ear. By far the most common of these is seborrhoeic dermatitis of the scalp, which produces excessive dandruff. Extreme irritation results, which is worse in hot weather and is increased by bathing. This condition often also affects the back of the ears causing painful cracks at the top and bottom of the junction of the auricle with the head. Scratching causes invasion of the skin and meatal wall by bacteria. The bacteriology is often mixed. *Pseudomonas pyocyaneas* is commonly found. Staphylococci are secondary invaders.

Treatment. The scalp is treated with frequent shampoos with spirit soap and the application of lotions or ointment prescribed by a skin specialist. For the ear condition, meticulous toilet is essential. Treatment can only be adequately carried out by trained personnel — the patient cannot be trusted to do it. Hence, nursing is important. The meatus must be gently mopped right down to the drum under direct vision. Then the appropriate medication is applied. There may be daily packing, with, for example, 8% aluminium acetate or glycerine and ichthyol. Later, neomycin and hydrocortisone ointments are often used. (N.B. Antibiotics are used only with steroids.) Drops are applied when the skin is almost healed.

Eczema of the ear

Eczema is a sensitization dermatitis characterized by the formation of vesicles which rupture and discharge a serous fluid. This exudate either dies and forms pinhead crusts or a continuous oozing occurs. As the inflammatory reaction dies down, the exudate ceases and the skin becomes covered with small scales. This sequence of events may last several weeks or years and the disease may be arrested for long periods.

Treatment. An eczema is generally due to allergy or to chemical irritation, and the patient is usually treated generally. The local treatment consists of cleanliness, the relief of irritation and the avoidance of scratching. A useful application to help in relief and healing is a paint containing gentian violet. The external meatus should be swabbed with this solution and then dried by means of a blower.

Herpes simplex and herpes zoster

Both these conditions occasionally affect the outer ear and are treated as other forms of otitis externa.

Herpes zoster is an acute inflammation of the sensory ganglion of a cutaneous nerve and is characterized by groups of vesicles which last for one to two weeks and then dry, leaving scarred areas. It can occur on the fifth and seventh cranial nerves — the Gasserian and geniculate ganglia. The disease is marked by severe pain and irritation which may persist for many months after the skin lesion has healed.

Furunculosis

Boils commonly arise in the cartilaginous portion of the external auditory meatus, and like boils elsewhere arise as staphylococcal infections of the hair follicles. They are often secondary to seborrhoeic dermatitis. They may develop into abscesses.

Symptoms. There is severe pain owing to the unyielding texture of the tissues. The pain is felt in the front of the ear (as distinct from mastoid pain, which is behind), which is tender on manipulation. Swelling of the meatus produces obstructive deafness. As each boil 'points' and discharges its contents, there is a remission of pain, but fresh boils tend to arise.

Treatment. Systemic treatment with an antibiotic is usually commenced at the onset of the condition. The pain may be relieved to some extent by the application of heat. Where the meatus is swollen, gauze wicks soaked in warm glycerin and 10% ichthyol may be gently packed into the auditory canal and a thermal pad applied outside. For recurrent boils, vaccine therapy is sometimes used.

Aspergillosis (otomycosis)

This is a fungoid infection which attacks the external auditory meatus. It produces a membrane looking rather like damp blotting paper covered with black or yellow spots. The patient complains of irritation and discharge.

The treatment commonly employed is the application of nystatin or gentian violet. Oils and ointments must not be applied to the ear, since these encourage the growth of the fungus.

Other fungi may cause otomycosis. Griseofulvin taken internally is now used as treatment.

Haematoma of the auricle

This unsightly condition is caused by injury, particularly from a blow on the ear as in boxing. Small bruises require no treatment as a rule, but a large haematoma, besides being painful owing to the retention of blood in dense tissues that cannot swell easily, is in danger of becoming infected. Infection commonly leads to the destruction of cartilage.

Treatment of a large haematoma. The pinna is first cleaned, using swabs dipped in methylated spirit. The haematoma is then aspirated, using a hypodermic syringe and needle, with full aseptic technique. A dressing is then firmly bandaged in position.

Alternatively, the Elastoplast technique may be employed. This consists of cleaning the ear, aspirating the blood-stained contents of the haematoma, filling the hollows of the pinna with a mould of Stent's compound or sponge rubber and securing this with Elastoplast. The strapping is laid on both sides of the auricle and the edges are stuck to each other. The surplus is then trimmed to make a neat dressing. This is left for ten days. If necessary, the aspiration is repeated.

Excess of wax in the ear

The normal cerumen secreted in the auditory meatus occasionally accumulates in the lower corner of the meatus against the ear drum and may interfere with hearing. This usually happens in persons suffering from some degree of seborrhoeic dermatitis. The mass contains flakes of epithelial debris. This is usually removed by careful syringing, by a doctor or a member of the nursing staff who has undergone the appropriate training. But, if the eardrum is known to be perforated, syringing should not be carried out, owing to the danger of fluid entering the middle ear and setting up inflammation. Instead, the wax is picked out by the doctor, using a sharp hook.

Foreign bodies in the ear

It is most important that amateur attempts to remove a hard foreign body from the ear should be discouraged, especially with a sharp instrument which may damage the eardrum. Owing to the curves of the external auditory meatus, it is easier to push an object into an inaccessible part of the canal than to withdraw it. Sometimes, however, an insect such as a fly or a spider may find its way into an ear, and an attempt to remove it should be made. A fly buzzing inside one's ear makes a thunderous roar, most alarming to a child and quite disturbing to an adult. A little warm water inserted into the meatus from a teaspoon may float out the insect. If this is not effective, spirit drops should be instilled to kill the insect, which is then syringed out. A vegetable object such as a pea should not be treated by syringing, because, if the procedure fails to remove it, the pea will swell, become impacted and will be more difficult to remove. Mineral objects, such as beads, can often be syringed out, but if this is unsuccessful, the surgeon will use aural forceps or a sharp hook in a strong reflected light. On rare occasions, an incision behind the auricle is necessary to remove the object.

Irritation caused by discharge sometimes explains why a child inserts foreign bodies into the ear. Obstruction of drainage may follow, giving rise to severe symptoms of sepsis.

Rupture of the eardrum

This may be the result of a blow over the external meatus or from bomb explosions or gunfire, or may be due to fracture of the skull. Whatever the cause, even if there is bleeding from the ear, the only treatment should be to apply a sterile gauze dressing and give an antibiotic to prevent infection. If suppuration should follow the rupture, then the patient is treated for acute otitis media.

Exostosis of the ear

Bony outgrowths occasionally arise from the wall of the external auditory meatus. They are usually single but may be multiple, and the bone composing them is much more dense than that of the meatus.

If large, they cause obstructive deafness, and will complicate the treatment of otitis externa. Wax may accumulate.

Removal is difficult owing to the hardness of the exostosis and its common position in the posterior meatal wall, in close relation with the facial nerve and other important structures. If an operation is considered necessary, the approach may be either through the meatus or behind the ear.

New growths of the outer ear

Rodent ulcer and squamous epitheliomata are comparatively common in the outer ear. A rodent ulcer arises on the auricle; an epithelioma may develop on the concha or in the external meatus. On the concha it is of the ulcerative type; in the meatus it is sessile or papillomatous.

Treatment. Small ulcers on the concha may be treated by excision or the application of a radium plaque. Growths in the external meatus require excision of the whole cartilaginous meatus. When the growth is near the drum, radical mastoidectomy is often advisable in order to remove a safe margin of bone and epithelium. This is usually combined with irradiation.

6 Diseases of the middle ear

Acute otitis media

Infection of the middle ear almost always travels from the naso-pharynx via the pharyngotympanic tube (Eustachian tube). The presence of adenoids and the wider, straighter pharyngotympanic tube of childhood both favour this passage of infection. Otitis media is particularly common after infections of the upper respiratory tract — for example, influenza, scarlet fever, measles and diphtheria. It sometimes follows swimming in public baths, but often inflammation following such exercise is due to micro-organisms already present in the nose and throat. The organisms responsible for otitis media are the haemolytic *Streptococcus pyogenes*, *Streptococcus viridans*, staphylococci and pneumococci. Any infection may lead to bone destruction and intracranial complications.

In the early stages of inflammation, the mucous membrane of the middle ear is reddened, then it exudes serous fluid which collects in the cavity. The infection spreads to the mastoid aircells and if not released the exudate soon becomes purulent.

Signs and symptoms. At first the patient notices slight deafness and popping noises in the ear. These are quickly succeeded by pain and the condition rapidly becomes worse. Pain and deafness are the prominent symptoms. There may be tinnitus (noises in the ear) of a pulsating nature, but this is not usually severe. The pain is more severe at night. There may be tenderness over the mastoid process. An infant suffering from acute otitis media will be fretful and restless, rubbing his hand over his ear and his head in the pillow. The temperature is usually raised and may reach 39.5°C (103°F) or 40°C (104°F) in children. On examination, the eardrum is seen to be flushed, with a network of dilated blood vessels. At a very early stage of inflammation, the malleus is still visible. In a few hours the membrane is bulging and bright red and the malleus is obscured. If the inflammation is untreated, a yellow spot appears in front of or behind the handle of the malleus, rupture follows and blood-stained pus escapes into the meatus. Pain is then relieved as a rule. If it persists, the indication is probably the retention of pus in the mastoid process. The patient is often not admitted to hospital, but an increasing deafness accompanying otitis media must be regarded as a grave sign.

Treatment. This turns upon the severity of the condition on the one hand and the stage it has reached on the other. In a mild case, the doctor may decide that all that are needed are such simple remedies as a mild analgesic and local heat.

Where the patient is ill and whether the drum has ruptured or not, an antibiotic is given and an analgesic is prescribed for the pain. If the drum has ruptured, a sterile dressing is kept over the ear (see Fig. 6.1), and the discharge is dry mopped out two to three times daily.

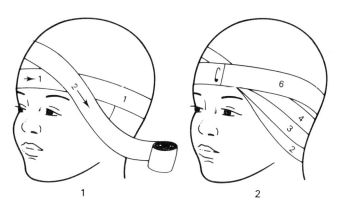

Fig. 6.1. *Applying a bandage to the ear.*

The patient is usually kept in bed. The accompanying nasal infection is treated by steam inhalations, etc.

The operation of myringotomy (incision of the eardrum) is mainly reserved for those conditions where fluid continues to accumulate in the tympanum after adequate antibiotic treatment, or where pain or deafness persists.

The nurse's duties in relation to these patients will be to give the antibiotics and other medicines, to change the ear dressings and to report any signs of complications such as mastoiditis or intracranial invasion by the infection.

Acute mastoiditis

This has become exceedingly rare and is usually seen in neglected cases of acute otitis media. The complication is indicated by an intensification of the symptoms. Pain becomes severe. Tenderness and usually redness and swelling occur behind the ear. In late cases, the swelling thrusts the auricle forward in a characteristic fashion. The amount of discharge usually increases, but may lessen temporarily. In infants, the bony outer wall of the mastoid is thin and may rupture, so that pus may escape and form an abscess beneath the skin.

Treatment. Intensive antibiotic therapy may still check the infection in the early stage before breakdown of bone and abscess formation have occurred, but the patient must be kept under close observation. The operation of mastoidectomy is usually needed.

Chronic otitis media

The change from acute otitis to the chronic form is ill-defined, but the term 'chronic suppurative otitis media' is applied when there is suppuration of long standing with no signs of acute inflammation. Pain is usually absent.

The *discharge* varies from thin mucopurulent secretion to offensive, cheesy material which escapes into the external meatus through a perforation in the eardrum. If scanty it may even escape the patient's notice! The odour is dependent upon secondary infection due to obstructed drainage. The nature of the discharge helps to indicate the primary source of the otitis. Mucoid discharge is characteristic of a primary post-nasal infection, spreading by the pharyngotympanic tube into the lower part of the middle ear. A thick offensive discharge indicates bony disease in the attic or mastoid bone. The site of the disease is indicated by the position of the perforation (see Fig. 6.2). Frequently attic perforations can be seen, but in some cases the discharge is so scanty that it dries over a perforation and obscures it. In these cases, the discharge becomes foul-smelling, and cholesteatoma is suspected. Blood-stained discharge indicates granulation tissue and polypi which in turn point to deep-seated disease of bone.

Deafness in some degree, from slight impairment to complete absence of hearing, accompanies chronic otitis media.

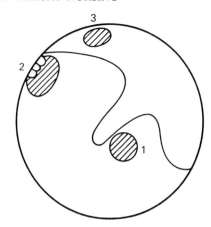

Fig. 6.2. *Perforations of the ear-drum. 1. Central. 2. Marginal, with granulations. 3. Attic perforation, which is associated with choleste-atoma.*

Granulations are bright red, sessile masses. They bleed readily, and can be touched by a probe without producing pain. A polypus does not differ materially from granulation tissue. It is attached by a stalk and, being covered with squamous epithelium, does not bleed when touched, but it may obscure the details of the drum.

Secretory otitis media ('glue ear')

This is a condition seen with increasing frequency during recent years. A clear exudate fills the middle ear and the tympanic membrane often has a yellowish tinge. The patient complains of stuffiness in the ear. It is due to a dysfunction of the pharyngo-tympanic tube following repeated acute attacks of infection or obstruction (e.g. from adenoids) or alterations in air pressure such as occur when landing in an aircraft. In all these cases, air cannot enter the middle ear from the tube, and middle ear effusion often results.

Treatment. In children, nasal decongestants may be prescribed. If this fails to cure the condition a myringotomy and insertion of grommets will be carried out in theatre. For adults, pharyngo-tympanic tube catheterization or myringotomy with insertion of a drain is necessary. If drainage is inadequate, fibrous adhesions may bind the ossicles, retracting the tympanic membrane and causing conductive or adhesive deafness and eventually cholesteatoma formation. In severe cases, this leads to the necessity for a hearing aid.

Cholesteatoma

This is a yellowish-grey mass consisting of epithelial tissue, pus and crystals of cholesterin. It occurs in the middle ear and may be either the cause or the result of chronic suppuration, according to its origin. It may be formed in various ways:

1. As an aberration of development, squamous epithelium being included in other tissues. This form may occur within the cranial cavity.
2. As a result of inflammation, by destruction of the edge of the drum and the ingrowth of epithelium from the external meatus. Constant desquamation of epithelial cells forms a mass which erodes bone. It may destroy the whole of the middle and inner ear and even constitute an intracranial tumour. In the middle ear it is liable to keep up an infection and lead to serious intracranial complications.
3. The character of the epithelium in the middle ear changes from ciliated to stratified epithelium as a result of infection.

Spread of infection from the middle ear

A backward spread of infection from the middle ear will penetrate:

1. The mastoid air cells. This is commonly concurrent with otitis media.
2. The lateral sinus, further back.
3. The cerebellum, still further back.

An inward spread will reach the inner ear, causing labyrinthitis.

An upward spread will involve the temporal lobe of the brain, leading to meningitis, cerebral abscess and other intracranial complications.

COMPLICATIONS OF MIDDLE EAR DISEASE

All of these are becoming more rare and occur usually in acute exacerbations of chronic ear infections.

Lateral sinus thrombosis

Venous infection with thrombosis occurs first in a tributary vein and spreads quickly into the lateral sinus, part of which projects into the mastoid process, so that its wall easily becomes infected and adherent to the bone. This may lead to abscesses around the sinus (perisinous abscess). These are not uncommon in children. Should the sinus itself become inflamed, the very serious condition of thrombosis may develop. Particles of septic clot may be broken off into the blood stream and produce pyaemia (abscesses forming in other parts of the body), or the patient may develop septicaemia.

Signs. Sinus thrombosis follows two main types:

1. The acute, fulminating type, which is typically shown by rigors or convulsions in infancy, and a persistently swinging temperature.
2. The commoner form, in which the ear continues to discharge and there are unexplained spikes of pyrexia. The infection occasionally spreads down the jugular vein. The sternomastoid muscle is painful and tender. The patient is well orientated and there is no headache unless the infection spreads to the meninges.

Diagnosis of thrombosis is made by Queckenstedt's test. For this purpose a lumbar puncture is performed, and the jugular vein of the affected side is compressed. If this causes no rise of pressure in the spinal fluid, obstruction is present at a higher level.

Treatment. The ear condition will probably indicate the need for a mastoid operation. When this has been completed the bone over the sinus (if not destroyed by the disease) is removed, the lateral sinus is incised and the clot removed. Bleeding is controlled by the insertion of gauze packing between the sinus and the bone.

In dressing the mastoid wound, the gauze packing (unless of the absorbable variety) should be removed gradually, 2–3 cm each day, in order to avoid bleeding, which would probably occur should the packing be removed suddenly.

Antibiotics should be continued until after the symptoms have subsided.

INTRACRANIAL COMPLICATIONS OF OTITIS

By means of septic thrombi carried in the blood stream, infection from the middle or inner ear can spread into the cranium. It may pass directly through the thin bone which forms the roof of the middle ear, or through the petrous bone or through anatomical channels between the ear and the brain, for example, through the labyrinth by the internal auditory meatus. A diffuse meningitis may follow, or the infection may be localized into an abscess. The abscess may be between the dura and the bone (extradural) or within the dura (subdural) or in the brain substance itself.

Meningitis

Signs and symptoms. With the onset of meningitis, fever becomes higher, there is restlessness and loss of appetite. Meningeal irritation is first shown by discomfort on flexing the head forward and photophobia with generalized headache. This is followed by severe headache and rigidity of the neck. There are increased deep reflexes and characteristic changes in the cerebrospinal fluid — notably a decrease in carbohydrate and an increased cell count. Bacteria may be grown by culture of the fluid. As the intracranial pressure rises, other symptoms appear, such as vomiting, insomnia, a relatively slow pulse rate and Cheyne–Stokes respiration. The patient lies on his back with his eyes closed, in a stupor from which he may not be easily roused.

The diagnosis is established by lumbar puncture, which should be performed on the earliest suspicion of meningitis. The meningitis complicating otitis media is usually due to streptococci, staphylococci or pneumococci. The last was once considered to be the most serious, but the prognosis has been improved with modern antibiotic regimens. Nowadays the most dangerous infections are those that are less sensitive to antibiotics and the sulpha drugs, for example, *Proteus vulgaris* (varieties of which are commonly responsible for epidemic enteritis) and *Haemophilus influenzae*. Sulpha preparations find their way into the cerebrospinal fluid. Some antibiotics, e.g. penicillin, do not.

Treatment. When the causative organism is found, the appropriate preparation is given. Sulpha drugs are given in full doses orally (or intravenously if there is vomiting). Antibiotics are given intramuscularly or intravenously. Free drainage of the primary source of infection is combined with repeated lumbar puncture. Dehydration must be avoided and intravenous fluid is often required. A patient with meningitis is very ill and needs much patience and attention from his nurses, together with careful observation and recording of all vital signs. He may be irrational, irritable or delirious and the nurse will need all her tact to carry out the necessary care of mouth, pressure areas, and feeding. A sedative is often given before attempting lumbar puncture.

Intracranial abscesses

Extradural abscess

Extradural abscess, which is rarely diagnosed before operation, as it is part of a mastoid abscess, gives no special symptoms beyond those of mastoid infection. Necrosis of bone in the mastoid area reaches the middle, or sometimes the posterior cranial fossa, where the dura mater reacts by thickening and closing off the infection. Unless the abscess is drained, the infection may penetrate the dura mater and other meninges, causing first a stage of encephalitis and then abscess of the brain tissue.

Cerebral abscess

A cerebral abscess is most commonly situated in the temporal lobe. The mode of spread is usually by a septic thrombophlebitis. The abscess is at first thin-walled and poorly shut off; later, it becomes thick-walled.

Symptoms. Headache, vomiting, giddiness and slowness of speech and thought are the general symptoms. In the early stages, the temperature and pulse rates may be raised in response to the sepsis, but as the compression of the brain increases, the temperature becomes subnormal and the pulse slow. Weakness of certain muscles may indicate to the doctor the position of the abscess. Lumbar puncture is performed only with the greatest caution, lest sudden alteration in pressure cause harm. If the cerebrospinal fluid is examined it is found to have fewer chlorides and more protein than normal. Should the abscess be leaking into the ventricles or the subarachnoid space, the fluid will be turbid.

An abscess in the left temporal lobe of a right-handed patient produces aphasia — the inability to name common objects although the patient can describe them.

Eye changes may accompany cerebral abscess.

Cerebellar abscess

A cerebellar abscess in the posterior cranial fossa causes symptoms of cerebral infection and raised intracranial pressure as previously described. The localizing symptoms are a varying nystagmus (oscillation of the eyeball) and loss of muscular co-ordination.

Treatment of brain abscess

The nursing treatment is very important as the patient may be unconscious or disorientated and may be incontinent. He may need nasal feeding or intravenous therapy. The diagnostic treatment will be lumbar puncture, and encephalography or arteriography. Surgical treatment is carried out by a neurosurgeon. Generally burr holes are made, the abscess is tapped and the cavity is filled with antibiotic. This is repeated whenever signs of raised intracranial pressure occur again until the abscess has contracted to a small unimportant scar. The abscess may be dissected out if it fails to contract satisfactorily.

The primary ear condition is treated when the neurosurgeon thinks the patient is fit for this.

Facial paralysis of otitic origin

The facial nerve may be involved by an infection of the mastoid bone cells surrounding the facial canal, or may be damaged during operation.

As the facial nerve supplies the muscles of expression, complete paralysis is shown by marked asymmetry of the face, the affected side being devoid of its natural folds and expression. Any attempt at smiling causes the face to be drawn to the opposite side. The patient cannot raise the eyebrow or close the eye or show his teeth on the paralysed side. He cannot whistle or pronounce the labial consonants. Paralysis of the buccinator muscle allows food to collect between the gum and the cheek. The chorda tympani branch of the facial nerve may be damaged, resulting in loss of taste and a diminished salivary secretion.

Facial paralysis also occurs without apparent cause and without ear disease. These ideopathic types are known as Bell's palsy.

Treatment:

1. *Before operation.* If signs of facial paralysis appear early in the course of an acute middle ear infection, they will usually disappear with antibiotic treatment. In the established case of otitis media, operation and decompression of the nerve via the mastoid is usually needed.
2. *During operation.* Should the nerve be damaged during operation, it is immediately sutured.
3. *After operation.* If the paralysis is noticed soon after operation, but is incomplete, recovery is likely. If it is complete, the operation cavity will probably need to be reopened and the nerve explored. If the paralysis develops a few days after operation, it will almost certainly recover.

   After section of the nerve and grafting, recovery usually takes about 12 months, and then the movements of the facial muscles are not perfect. The patient is usually provided with a splint to raise the corner of the mouth and so avoid over-stretching the cheek muscles. Especial care must be taken to ensure oral cleanliness as the patient cannot wash out the mouth on the affected side. Since normal blinking does not occur on the affected side, the nurse should bathe the eye carefully. Sometimes the eyelids may need suturing to protect the cornea (tarsorrhaphy).
4. *Bell's palsy* usually responds to physiotherapy, but in certain circumstances the nerve may need to be decompressed as it lies in its bony canal in order to promote recovery.

Otosclerosis

This is a disease affecting the middle and inner ear and is at present of unknown origin. It causes progressive conductive deafness, commencing in youth. Females suffer more often than males, and there is a familial tendency. For some reason, perhaps metabolic, normal bone in the labyrinth is absorbed and a deposit of new vascular web-like bone appears in its place. There is usually more than one primary focus. The area around the oval window is most often first affected, less frequently the round window, but the condition slowly spreads through the labyrinth. In time this spongy bone becomes compact. Deafness occurs as soon as the windows cease to vibrate normally, and increases as the stapes becomes fixed. The patient commonly hears much better in a noise. She speaks in a typically soft voice, in contrast with the loud voice of a person with nerve deafness.

On examination, the ear drum appears normal. Tuning fork tests show a conductive deafness and, in older patients, some nerve deafness. There is no improvement in hearing after inflation of the pharyngotympanic tube, which is dry and clear.

Treatment. This is usually surgical. The stapes is removed completely and replaced by a prosthesis. Hearing aids can be supplied if the patient is elderly or does not wish for operation or if there is too much internal ear damage.

7 Diseases of the inner ear

Disease of the inner ear produces dizziness due to disturbance of the fluid levels in the semicircular canals of the labyrinth or of the function of the auditory nerve, or both. Deafness resulting from disease of the inner ear occurs in varying degrees, but hearing is never completely lost unless the cochlea or the auditory nerve is destroyed.

Inner ear deafness

Inner ear deafness may be congenital or acquired.

Causes of congenital inner ear deafness

1. Maldevelopment of the ear. Essential parts may be absent.
2. Congenital syphilis.
3. Disease of the mother during pregnancy. Rubella (German measles), in particular, is held responsible for a defect in the cochlear mechanism.
4. Rhesus factor antibodies in the mother's blood.

Causes of acquired inner ear deafness

1. Labyrinthitis. This may be a non-suppurative effusion, usually in one ear only, following mumps. Cerebrospinal meningitis may cause bilateral inflammation of the labyrinth which is often permanent.
2. Concussion. A blow or explosion without obvious injury to the structure of the ear may cause destruction of the auditory nerve endings.
3. Occupation. Exposure to percussive noises in certain occupations may result in permanent damage to hearing. This can be prevented by wearing the protective ear-muffs normally supplied by the employer.
4. Old age. Senile deafness is due to the degeneration of the

auditory nerve. There is often an atrophy of part of the membranous cochlea causing loss of hearing for high notes. The deafness is usually bilateral and is not accompanied by tinnitus.

Deafness in infancy

This condition may be inherited or congenital, due to maldevelopment or intrauterine disease affecting the ear, but deafness may be acquired at a very early age, e.g. from meningitis, and this will prevent the child from learning to speak. The child requires careful training in lip reading, and a transistor hearing aid. The latter may be supplied to babies in cots, and its early use can lead to the accurate development of speech. If the hearing loss is severe, special educational methods will be needed.

Tests of vestibular function

Disease of the vestibule causes three main symptoms:

1. Vertigo.
2. Nausea and vomiting — these are called 'visceral reflexes'.
3. Nystagmus.

Tests are used to stimulate the labyrinth in various ways, comparisons being made between the reactions of the two ears in order to discover the presence of abnormality. The common tests are the caloric test and the rotation test.

The caloric test

This depends on convection currents produced in the semicircular canals by heating or cooling a portion of the labyrinth. The flow of endolymph stimulates specialized nerve endings causing giddiness and nystagmus. Since cold produces a greater response than heat, cold water is used first. If the drum is perforated, air may be introduced instead of water.

The apparatus required includes an aural syringe; a receiver; a jug of cold water at 30°C (86°F), i.e. 7°C below body temperature; protective sheeting; a vomit bowl; and a stop watch.

The patient lies on his back, and his head is raised 30°, which brings his lateral semicircular canals into the vertical position. The receiver is placed below the ear which is to be tested. The doctor fills the aural syringe with cold water, straightens out the external auditory canal and places the nozzle of the syringe into the canal. The patient (whose clothing is protected by the sheeting) is advised by the doctor to fix his eyes on a spot immediately in front of him. The nurse advises the doctor when to commence the flow of water. After 40 seconds the nurse will indicate to the doctor to cease the flow of water, which is returned into the receiver. If no nystagmus occurs, the test may be repeated using water at 20°C (68°F). The normal duration of the nystagmus is two minutes. With loss of function, it will be less or may not appear at all.

Some patients are nauseated after the test and may require to be left lying flat for some time.

The rotation test

The patient sits in a rotating chair. Rotation of the chair with the patient holding his head in varying positions will produce nystagmus of varying character and duration. Both ears are affected at the same time but in opposite directions. The correct interpretation of the test is difficult. The tendency to fall is away from the affected labyrinth, but the patient may make such an effort to recover that he falls the other way.

The duration of the nystagmus is noted in seconds. If no nystagmus is produced, the labyrinth is assumed to be functionless.

More accurate methods are involved in what is called electronystagmography. This allows accurate measurement of the speed, amplitude and frequency of the nystagmus; these measurements can be more important than duration.

AURAL VERTIGO

As has been mentioned before, dizziness may occur in a large number of conditions concerned with the cardiovascular system. Vertigo whose origin is in the ear itself may be due to:

Obstruction of the pharyngo-
  tympanic tube.   } Disturbance of pressure in
Middle ear disease.   the middle ear may affect
                             the labyrinth.

Labyrinthitis: aural vertigo with suppuration.

Ménière's disease: a non-suppurative condition of the labyrinth causing paroxysmal attacks of vertigo.

Tumour in the course of the eighth cranial nerve, for example, a temporal lobe tumour or a cerebellar tumour.

It may also occur after stapedectomy and other ear operations for a few days.

Suppurative labyrinthitis

Suppurative labyrinthitis may follow otitis media or an injury to the ear. Circumscribed and diffuse types are described, but the difference is only one of degree. It usually follows chronic otitis media which is frequently due to cholesteatoma.

Symptoms

These are giddiness, especially on turning quickly or bending, loss of balance, nausea and vomiting. Nystagmus is present. On applying the caloric test, a diminished reaction is found in the affected ear. Hearing is fairly good as a rule, although it may fade, or the patient may be deaf from the original disease. If a fistula from the middle ear is present, then any sudden change in middle ear pressure will immediately produce acute labyrinthine reactions, provided that the labyrinth is functioning. The test is to exert sudden pressure on the tragus or to insert the nozzle of a Politzer bag into the external auditory meatus and apply suction or pressure.

Treatment

The patient should rest quietly in bed until the condition has stabilized. An antibiotic may be prescribed. When the symptoms have subsided, a mastoidectomy is performed. If there is total loss of hearing, it is wise to open the labyrinth. It may contain pus. Careful watch must always be made for meningitis.

Positional vertigo

The patient feels giddy only when his head is put in a certain position. If he is seen during an attack, nystagmus will be noticed.

Occasionally there is nausea, but there is no increase in deafness. The condition is usually due to a disturbance in the otolith apparatus of the semicircular canals and is self-limiting. The patient is often anxious and a tranquillizing drug may be prescribed.

Ménière's disease (paroxysmal aural vertigo)

This is a non-suppurative condition in which there is a hydrops distension of the membranous labyrinth, characterized by sudden vertigo in recurrent attacks associated with deafness and tinnitus. The deafness is very often pre-existent. It is perceptive and the caloric test shows diminished labyrinthine function.

Symptoms

The suddenness of the vertigo is the distinguishing feature of the condition. It may occur at night and waken the patient. Both ears may be affected. The giddiness is rotatory and, as a rule, in a definite direction. Both tinnitus and deafness are worse during the attack. As attacks become more frequent, deafness tends to persist and may become complete. Nystagmus is present during the paroxysms, but the patient's distress prevents full examination. The patient is quite helpless and incapacitated by the vertigo which may last a number of hours or days, and then passes off completely. At first, the attacks occur at long intervals and are comparatively slight, but their severity increases with their recurrence.

Treatment

In the acute attack, sodium phenobarbitone 60 to 200 mg, or chlorpromaxine hydrochloride (Largactil) is given by injection. It is of the utmost importance to reassure the patient that improvement will be achieved. He can be told that he is suffering from a definite disease — not 'merely from nerves'. The fear of an attack during traffic or work is liable to make him lose self-confidence and the nurse can do a great deal to improve his morale. The underlying cause of the attacks can be explained to most patients.

In the established case, a sedative such as 30 mg of phenobarbitone is given three times a day. Nicotinic acid up to 300 mg daily and restricted salt and fluid help control most patients satisfactorily. However, relapses are common.

Should dietetic and sedative treatment not be effective, an operation may be decided upon. The labyrinth on the affected side may be destroyed in various ways. The power of compensation in a labyrinthine mechanism is very great. If one is destroyed, the surviving labyrinth assumes control, and in a few weeks, giddiness ceases. Any hearing that the patient may have had in that ear is lost.

Recently, the use of ultrasound directed selectively at the semicircular canals of the affected side has been used. This is done via a Schwartze mastoid approach using special apparatus. The preoperative hearing is usually retained.

Vestibular neuronitis

This type of vertigo occurs in younger patients than does Ménière's disease. It is probably consequent on infective conditions of the nose and throat or may be caused by a virus infection. The nature of the attack is similar to Ménière's disease. Recurrent attacks are unlikely. Antihistamine drugs are helpful in its control.

Acoustic neuroma

This is a neurofibroma of the auditory nerve. The symptoms are similar to Ménière's disease, so diagnosis is not an easy matter. The otologist will usually refer the patient to a neurosurgeon for treatment.

8 Operations on the ear

Preoperative treatment

Ear operations in this country are nearly always performed under general anaesthesia. The local preparation requires the shaving of the head and neck for about 5 cm around the auricle. The remaining hair may be washed and must be fastened securely away from the operation site. If the operation is for treatment of acute infection, the patient has a considerable amount of tenderness and the shaving is occasionally done after the patient is anaesthetized. If not, it must be done gently, care being taken that the razor blade is sharp. The pinna and the meatus should be mopped clean and may be syringed. The skin is cleaned with spirit and perhaps some antiseptic of the surgeon's choice.

Myringotomy

This minor operation is carried out for acute otitis or for secretory otitis media. It is usually carried out under general anaesthesia through an aural speculum, or a Zeiss operating microscope may be used. A curved incision is made in the eardrum by means of a bayonet-shaped myringotome. In acute conditions an immediate escape of discharge follows, and this is mopped away with a gauze strip. A swab is sent to the laboratory, to discover the organisms present and their sensitivity. After operation the ear should be inspected frequently to ensure that the opening is adequate and the drainage free.

In secretory otitis, the discharge does not escape. As much as possible is removed by suction and a Teflon tube drain or 1 or 2 grommets are inserted.

Schwartze's operation or cortical mastoidectomy

Here a curved incision is made approximately 1.3 cm behind the auricular groove and is carried down to the bone, exposing the tip of the mastoid process. The mastoid cells and antrum are then removed with a gouge or dental burr. The cavity can be left wide open and allowed to granulate, or the wound may be stitched and a drain inserted. The drain is removed when the doctor issues the instruction to do so, normally once drainage has ceased. The stitches are removed on about the fifth day. An antibiotic is normally prescribed.

Radical mastoidectomy for chronic disease of the ear

By this operation the middle ear and the mastoid antrum are converted into a single cavity, two ossicles and part of the external auditory canal being removed. The posterior superior wall of the attic is removed, together with the malleus and incus. The cavity is curetted and made smooth, and all loose pieces of bone are washed out. Care is taken to avoid the lateral sinus, the facial nerve and the semicircular canals, also dislocation of the stapes, as this would open up a path into the labyrinth, into which infection might travel. The meatus is enlarged by means of specially designed flaps and the cavity is packed lightly with, for example, calcium alginate and penicillin or ribbon gauze soaked in bismuth, iodoform and paraffin paste (BIPP). As a rule, the post-auricular wound is sutured.

In some cases, after seven to ten days, the cavity in the bone is covered with a skin graft taken from behind the ear.

Modified radical mastoidectomy

The posterosuperior wall of the external auditory meatus is resected, but an attempt is made to conserve as much of the eardrum and ossicles as possible. The wound drains through the meatus.

Tympanoplasty

Between the cortical and radical operations there is now a whole range of operations designed to eradicate chronic disease in the middle ear and mastoid, while at the same time reconstructing a more or less effective sound-conducting mechanism. These operations are sometimes done end-aurally (see below) or from behind. Important principles are to put some form of graft in connection with the ossicles and to close the perforation in the drum membrane. Temporalis fascia is generally used.

This work is carried out under a Zeiss operating microscope. It will be one of the duties of the theatre nurse to familiarize herself with this instrument and to be able to adjust it.

End-aural operations

In recent years, operations using a different approach to the ear have been performed. Instead of using a post-auricular incision (Fig. 8.1), these operations enter the ear through an incision in front of the ear through the concha into the meatus (Fig. 8.2). By using this route,

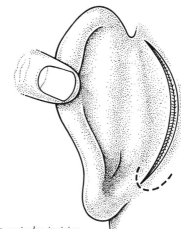

Fig. 8.1. *Post-auricular incision.*

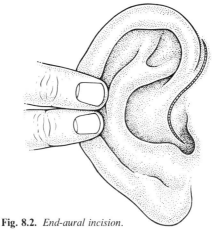

Fig. 8.2. *End-aural incision.*

exostoses of the external auditory meatus may be removed without damaging the healthy mastoid process, and in certain cases, a mastoidectomy for treatment of infection can be more satisfactorily performed. Pathological tissue can be clearly seen and removed.

Pre-operative treatment

In addition to the procedure outlined at the beginning of this chapter, a course of antibiotic therapy is commenced the day before operation.

Postoperative treatment

The patient is nursed in the most comfortable position. He may get up as soon as he is able. Dimenhydrinate (Dramamine) 25–50 mg is given as necessary to allay giddiness. Antibiotic therapy is continued for a five-day course. Any pack is removed on the first day and any drainage tubes on the second day. The dressing is changed and the sutures removed on the fifth day. The patient may be discharged from hospital once the sutures are removed. He is given an out-patient clinic appointment to return within two weeks. It is important for the nurse to note and report any facial weakness that the patient may show. This may be due to pressure from the pack. It can be relieved easily before irreparable damage is done.

THE SURGERY OF OTOSCLEROTIC DEAFNESS

Stapes mobilization

This is carried out under general anaesthesia, using a speculum and Zeiss operating microscope. The eardrum is reflected, and the stapes is exposed and gently rocked so as to mobilize it and re-establish the vibration of the oval window.

Stapedectomy

Usually the mobilization fails. In such a case, the stapes is deliberately dislocated and its crura fractured. The oval window is re-established by removal of bone and an artificial stapes is inserted. This consists either of a fat graft on a stainless steel wire, or alternatively of a very small stainless steel or plastic piston clamped to the incus. The eardrum is replaced and the ear packed for a day.

The advantages of these two operations are the short stay in hospital and the ultimately normal ear passage.

The results of stapedectomy are excellent and generally only limited by the efficiency of the cochlea.

Postoperative treatment

This is as for tympanoplasty (p. 57), but the patient is nursed on the unaffected side for 24 hours. After 48 hours he may sit out of bed for a few minutes, but care must be taken as his power of balance may take some time to recover. When this is satisfactory, he is allowed home. There may be some loss of taste on one side, but this is transient. Patients are told not to blow their nose sharply.

Labyrinthectomy for Ménière's disease

After opening the mastoid antrum and exposing the horizontal semicircular canal, the bony wall is burred out. Thereafter, the membranous canal is deliberately picked up with a fine hook and destroyed. Inasmuch as the middle ear is not opened, the cavity can be closed, and healing occurs by first intention. The patient's vertigo is usually cured, but any residual hearing in that ear is sacrificed.

The postoperative treatment follows closely that of stapedectomy. The patient should be warned that a slight residual dizziness will persist for some days after operation. Usually he is allowed out of bed within a week and is given special head exercises. He may be discharged in two to three weeks and return to work in two months.

Alternatively, the membranous labyrinth can be reached with a permeatal approach to the oval window, as in stapedectomy. The membrane is again picked out on a hook and alcohol is injected.

It is very important that all post-operative dressings be performed aseptically, either in the ward, a special dressing room or in the theatre.

9 Nursing techniques relating to the ear

Syringing of the ear

This procedure is dangerous in unskilled hands, because of the risk of the eardrum being perforated prior to the procedure, or as a result of the procedure.

A nurse should never syringe an ear, even on instructions from a doctor, unless she has undergone supervised practice. If deemed competent to perform the procedure, the nurse will have a written statement of authorization from her employing authority.

If the procedure is being performed to remove an accumulation of wax in the ear, drops of warm sodium bicarbonate, or any other solution with a similar action, should be inserted for a day or two prior to the procedure. Sodium bicarbonate saponifies the wax, so that it washes out easily.

Requirements

1. An aural syringe with a removable nozzle.
2. Head light, or head mirror, to reflect light from a lamp.
3. Lotion for syringing
   (a) Normal saline solution; or
   (b) Salt and sodium bicarbonate solution.
4. A lotion thermometer.
5. Aural forceps.
6. Dissecting forceps.
7. Fine wool swabs.
8. A kidney-shaped receiver for the returned lotion.
9. A paper bag for soiled swabs.
10. A receiver for soiled instruments.
11. Protective material for the patient's clothing.

The temperature of the lotion is very important. If it is much above or below body temperature, the patient will suffer from giddiness, or may faint. The lotion should be at a temperature of 38°C (100°F) in the jug, prior to commencing the procedure. The nurse should ensure that the syringe is working smoothly. An aseptic technique should always be used, in case there is a hidden perforation of the eardrum, or wound of the aural canal.

Method

The patient sits with the ear to be treated towards the operator. The patient's clothing is protected, and the nurse shows the patient how to hold the receiver against the cheek, under the ear. The operator puts on the head light, or the head mirror, and arranges the lamp so that the light can be reflected from the mirror. After washing and drying her hands, the operator attaches the nozzle to the syringe. The syringe is filled with the lotion, and the air expelled. With one hand, the operator draws the pinna upwards and slightly backwards to straighten the external meatus, and with the other hand she holds the syringe and directs the lotion first along the roof of the canal, then along its floor (see Figs. 9.1 and 9.2). When the irrigation is finished, the ear is gently dried using dressed aural forceps, and the used material is then dropped into the paper bag. When finished, the ear should be inspected to check for any damage or infection.

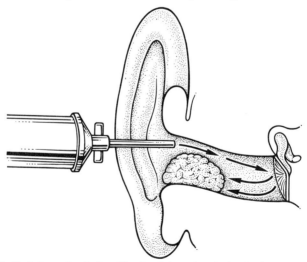

Fig. 9.1. *Technique of syringing. The tip of the syringe is just in the meatus and the jet of water is directed on to the posterior canal wall.*

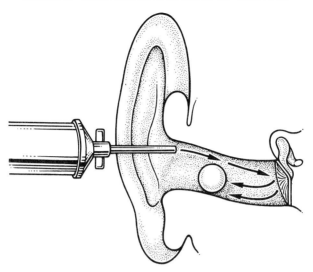

Fig. 9.2. *Removal of a foreign body.*

III The Nose and Accessory Sinuses

10 Anatomy of the nose
and paranasal sinuses

The nose is the first section of the respiratory passage, and extends from the roof of the mouth to the base of the skull and from the anterior to the posterior nares. It is divided into right and left nasal cavities by a septum, which is bony posteriorly but is composed of cartilage anteriorly. Air enters the nose through the nostrils (or anterior nares) and passes into the pharynx through the posterior nares.

For purposes of description the nose is divided into an external and an internal portion.

THE EXTERNAL NOSE

The external portion of the nose projects forwards from the centre of the face in a variety of shapes and sizes. The more or less pointed tip is called the *apex*, the part between the apex and the upper lip is the *base*. Where the nose joins the forehead is the *root* of the nose, and extending from the apex to the root is the *dorsum* of the nose, the portion nearest the root being called the bridge. The rounded eminence lateral to each nostril is called the wing of the nose, or the *ala nasi*.

The framework of the external nose is partly bone and partly cartilage. The aperture of the bony part of the external nose is, as seen in a skull, somewhat the shape of a heart upside down, being bounded by the maxillae in the lower two-thirds and by the two nasal bones in the upper one-third. The nasal bones are interposed between the frontal processes of the maxillary bones.

The cartilaginous portion of the framework of the external nose consists of five major cartilages — the right and left lower nasal cartilages (forming the apex of the nose), right and left upper nasal cartilages, and the septal cartilage interposed vertically between these cartilages so as to form almost the whole of the septum of the anterior part of the nasal cavity — and several small alar cartilages which lie behind the lower nasal cartilages and above the fibrofatty tissue of the alae nasi. The five major cartilages may be variously fused to one another and to the bones by the continuity of the perichondrium and periosteum. The anterior-inferior portion of the septum is freely movable; it is not formed by the septal cartilage but by the septal processes of the lower nasal cartilages and by the skin. The tip of the nose can, therefore, be pulled up, down and around.

Muscles and nerve supply of the external nose

Small slips of muscle arising from the *fascia* over the nasal bones and inserted into the skin between the eyebrows, produce transverse wrinkles over the bridge of the nose; others compress or dilate the nasal apertures. All these muscles are supplied by branches of the facial nerve, whereas the skin covering the external nose is supplied by branches of the trigeminal nerve.

The skin of the nose

Over the bony portion of the external nose the skin is thin, and since it rests upon loose subcutaneous tissue containing very little fat, it is freely movable. As it approaches the apex and base of the nose the skin becomes a little thicker, and the subcutaneous tissue is much denser, becoming fibrofatty in nature, which means that the skin loses its mobility. It also acquires many large, sebaceous glands, the openings of which in relation to the very fine hairs are readily seen.

Blood supply

The external nose is supplied by a rich arterial network from several sources. Passing on to the nose near its root is a branch of the ophthalmic artery (from the internal carotid). From the side comes a small branch of the internal maxillary artery (from the external carotid). Just above and just below the ala run branches of the facial artery. These arterial branches anastomose with one another and with their fellows from the opposite side. The veins draining this area end in the anterior facial and ophthalmic veins. There is some anastomosis here which may become significant should infection occur, since the ophthalmic vein drains into the cavernous sinus inside the skull.

There are lymphatic capillary networks in the skin and walls of the external nose, particularly dense at the apex, alae and root, and which drain into the submaxillary group of lymph nodes and anastomose with the lymphatics of the mucous membrane of the nasal fossae.

THE INTERNAL NOSE

The internal nose comprises the cavity, divided by the septum into a right and left nasal fossa. The shape of the fossa, seen from in front, is of a rather long and narrow right-angled triangle, with the right angle formed by the septum and the floor of the nose, and the superior angle blunted by the roof of the fossa (see Fig. 10.1). The shape of the fossa in sagittal section is shown in Fig. 1.1 (p. 4).

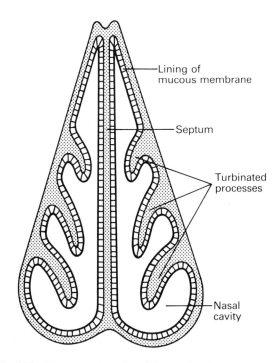

Lining of mucous membrane

Septum

Turbinated processes

Nasal cavity

Fig. 10.1. *Diagrammatic section of the nasal cavity.*

The anterior nares

The anterior nares (nostrils) are in the base of the nose. They vary a great deal in size, shape and the plane in which they lie, according to the individual and the race. Directly above each naris is a slightly expanded part of the fossa, called the vestibule. A recess of the vestibule extends forwards into the apex of the nose. The vestibule is lined by a thin skin which is tightly adherent to the underlying cartilage and fibrofatty tissue, and contains, in the lower part of the vestibule, coarse hairs which curve downward to guard the entrance. There are sebaceous glands related to these hairs.

The posterior nares

Each posterior naris is an oval opening measuring approximately 25 mm vertically and 10 mm transversely. It is completely bounded by bone covered with mucous membrane. Above it is the body of the sphenoid; medially is the posterior free margin of the vomer; laterally, the medial pterygoid plate of the sphenoid bone; and below, the posterior border of the horizontal portion of the palatal bone.

The roof of the nasal fossa

The roof of the nasal fossa is in the form of a narrow arch, the uppermost boundary being formed by the cribriform plate of the ethmoid bone (through which pass branches of the olfactory nerve), and the posterior sloping part by the body of the sphenoid, interrupted by the rounded orifice of the sphenoidal sinus.

The floor of the nose

The floor of the nose is approximately horizontal and is formed of bone — the anterior three-quarters by the palatine processes of the maxillae, and the posterior quarter by the horizontal processes of the palatine bones. The floor of each nasal fossa is slightly concave from side to side. Its width is, to some extent, dependent on the size of the maxillary sinus.

The nasal septum

The nasal septum is composed chiefly of a very thin plate of bone called the *vomer*, the perpendicular plate of the *ethmoid bone*, and the *septal cartilage*, described in relation to the external nose. Their relation to each other is shown in Fig. 10.2. In addition, small processes from the maxillae, the palatine bones, the sphenoid bone, the frontal bone and the nasal bones articulate with the three main constituents of the septum named above, and so contribute slightly to the margin of the septal framework.

Above the vestibule, the *lateral wall of the nasal fossa* presents three projections with a bony foundation which run more or less horizontally and diminish in length from the lowest to the highest. These are named the inferior, middle and superior concha or turbinate respectively. The portions of the nasal fossa overlapped by these conchae are called the inferior, middle and superior meatuses. The inferior concha is a separate bone which articulates with the

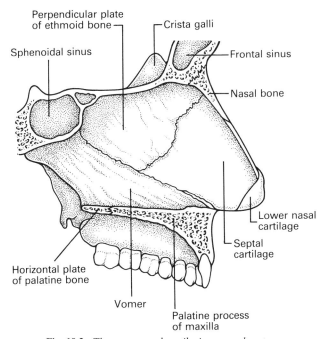

Fig. 10.2. *The osseous and cartilaginous nasal septum.*

maxilla, the lacrimal, the ethmoid and the palatine bones. The lacrimal duct which drains the secretion of the lacrimal gland from the conjunctival sac opens into the inferior meatus. Emotion stimulates the gland. As the duct is very small it cannot cope with a highly active gland, and if there is excessive secretion, this not only drains into the nose but also overflows down the cheeks as tears. A vigorous blowing of the nose can therefore sometimes prevent crying.

The middle and superior conchae are projections of the ethmoid bone. In the middle meatus are openings from the ethmoid air cells, the frontal sinus and the maxillary sinus. The superior meatus contains openings from the posterior ethmoid air cells. The sphenoid sinus opens into the 'sphenoethmoidal recess', which lies above and behind the superior concha.

The lining of the nose

The lining of the vestibule is composed of modified skin which merges into the mucous membrane which lines the nasal fossae proper. This nasal mucous membrane is of two kinds: olfactory and respiratory. Respiratory mucous membrane is discussed in Chapter 1. Olfactory mucous membrane is found in the upper part of the nose only — that is over the superior concha and the adjacent part of the septum. It has a yellowish tinge, and is of stratified epithelium, containing olfactory cells which receive the stimuli which give rise to the sense of smell. Processes from the olfactory cells bundle together to form the olfactory nerves, which pass through the cribriform plate of the ethmoid bone to end in the olfactory bulb.

Blood supply

The lining of the nasal fossae receives its blood supply from branches of the external and internal carotid arteries. Venous plexuses form a cavernous tissue inside the nose, especially on the inferior conchae and lower part of the septum. The blood drains into veins which more or less follow the arteries.

Lymph supply

Lymph vessels from the vestibule and the adjacent part of the nasal fossa, communicate with the vessels of the external nose and eventually drain into the submandibular group of the lymph nodes. There is some communication between the lymphatics of the right and left sides, particularly in the mobile septum. From the remaining part of the nasal fossa, the lymphatics run posteriorly and drain into the retropharyngeal and deep cervical glands. There is some connection between the lymphatics of the nasal fossa, through the cribriform plate of the ethmoid bone, with the subarachnoid space.

Nerve supply

Apart from the aforementioned olfactory nerves, which are distributed to the olfactory portion of the nasal mucous membrane, the nerves of the nasal fossa are branches of the trigeminal nerve. They are, for the most part, sensory fibres, but a few efferent fibres carry impulses to the glands and blood vessels in the lining of the nose.

THE ACCESSORY NASAL SINUSES

In the bones which help to form the framework of the nose are some important air spaces which communicate by relatively small openings with the nasal fossae. There are usually two (right and left) in the frontal bone, one in each maxillary bone, and two (right and left) in the sphenoid bone, called the *frontal*, *maxillary* and *sphenoid sinuses* respectively (see Fig. 10.3), while four to eight in each lateral mass of the ethmoid bone are called the *ethmoid air cells*.

The frontal sinuses

The frontal sinuses are usually located one on each side of the midline, where the part of the frontal bone that forms the forehead bends back to form the roofs of the orbits. They are separated from each other by a thin bony septum, which is usually deflected to the right or left, since the sinuses are not usually the same size and shape. Their average measurements are about 25 mm vertically, 18 mm transversely and 12 mm at the base, and their average capacity is 6 or 7 cm^3. They communicate with the middle meatus of the nasal cavity by a passage called the frontonasal duct. Occasionally there are several frontal sinuses, each with a duct into the nose. Either or both frontal sinuses may be missing. Sometimes they

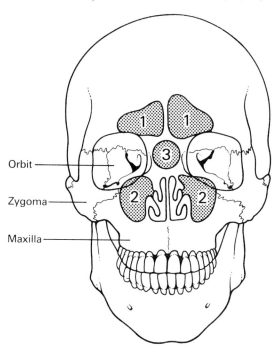

Fig. 10.3. *Diagrammatic view of the skull, showing the positions of the paranasal sinuses. 1. Frontal sinuses. 2 Maxillary sinuses, opening into the middle meati. 3. Sphenoid sinuses.*

extend deeply into the orbital portion of the frontal bone. Persons with large frontal sinuses very often, but not always, have prominent superciliary arches and to them may be ascribed (rightly or wrongly) great powers of concentration and intelligence, whereas the noble appearance of their foreheads is due to air, and not to brain!

The maxillary sinuses

The maxillary sinuses (or 'Antra of Highmore', as they are frequently called) are situated in the body and zygomatic process of each maxilla, but frequently extend into other processes of the bone. They are roughly pyramidal, their apexes formed by the zygomatic processes. Their floors are formed by the alveolar processes of the maxillae, and at their lowest are usually about 12 mm below the floor of the nasal fossa. The roofs of the sinuses form the floors of the orbits. Nerves to the upper teeth run in grooves or canals through the walls of the sinuses and contribute to their nerve supply. The extreme thinness of the walls of this cavity explains why a tumour arising in a sinus may project upwards into the orbit, forwards on to the cheek, downwards into the mouth or inwards to the nose. Many maxillary sinuses have inward bony projections in thin ridges, especially from their floor, making pockets which are difficult to drain (see Fig. 10.4).

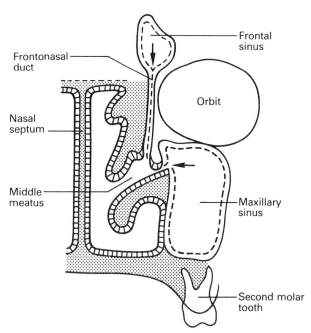

Fig. 10.4. *Drainage of frontal and maxillary sinus (note difficulty of drainage from the latter).*

The opening into the nasal fossa is usually high in the medial wall of the sinus and leads into the middle meatus. In many instances there is an additional opening lower in the wall, but this is generally closed by mucous membrane.

The sphenoid sinuses

The sphenoid sinuses lie in the body of the sphenoid bone and communicate with the nasal cavities through openings slightly above the level of the floors of the sinuses. The right sphenoid sinus is divided from the left one by an extremely thin bony septum, which is rarely central, so that they are not symmetrical. Like the other sinuses, they are not usually the same size, and their main development takes place after puberty. They are related above to the optic chiasma and the pituitary gland; on each side, to the internal carotid artery, the cavernous sinus and the third, fourth and fifth cranial nerves; in front, to the nerves and blood vessels crossing the roof of the nose to supply the nasal septum; behind, to the basilar artery and midbrain. It is interesting to note that the sphenoid sinus may be in relation to all three cranial fossae, and that the walls of the sinus may be extremely thin.

The ethmoidal sinuses

The ethmoidal sinuses consist of three groups of air cells, anterior, middle and posterior, which entirely occupy the lateral masses of the ethmoid bone and may extend into the neighbouring bones. The anterior and middle groups open into the middle meatus of the nose, and the posterior group into the superior meatus. The partitions between the air cells are very thin and sometimes missing — there may be an absence of bone between the anterior ethmoid cells and the lacrimal sac. Ethmoid cells which invade the roof of the orbit come into relationship with the anterior cranial fossa.

The paranasal sinuses begin to develop in fetal life, but are only minute spaces at birth. The frontal sinuses are fairly well developed at seven or eight years of age, but reach their full size after puberty. The maxillary sinuses reach full size after the eruption of permanent teeth.

11   Diseases of the nose

AFFECTIONS OF THE EXTERNAL NOSE

Diseases of the skin

Many who develop dermatitis or eczema of the nose suffer from the disease in other parts of the body also, and are treated in the skin wards and not in the Ear, Nose and Throat Unit. Some skin diseases, however, are especially associated with the nose and these will be considered here.

Acne rosacea

This condition is one of chronic hyperaemia of the face, particularly of the nose. There is a dilatation of blood vessels, with the formation of papules and pustules with core-like centres. In later stages there is permanent enlargement of the vessels and thickening of the connective tissue.

The cause may be dietary, alcohol or hot tea being especially liable to aggravate the disease. Gastrointestinal disturbances, emotion or the menopause may also be responsible. In all cases the main treatment is regulation of the diet. Stimulants and condiments should be avoided, also hot drinks and any articles of food found to give the patient indigestion.

Local applications with an astringent action, such as calamine, may be used. The lotion should be applied to the flushed area.

Furunculosis — boils

A boil is the result of inflammation of a hair follicle or sebaceous gland. There is suppuration and, after a few days, the expulsion of a mass of necrotic tissue, commonly known as the 'core'. The causative organism is commonly *Staphylococcus aureus*, which is often resistant to penicillin.

The furuncles occurring in the nose generally begin at the apex. There is at first deep-seated induration, which develops into a round, red, throbbing prominence, which becomes softer as suppuration occurs. The boil usually 'points' into the vestibule and its centre appears as a yellow spot. Until the core is discharged there is much pain, owing to the tightness of the skin over the nasal cartilages. There is frequently a recurrence, the site of the boil moving deeper into the nose.

With each boil there may be fewer obvious signs, but as there is less room for the skin to swell, the pain becomes more intense. The patient must be warned to resist the temptation to pick or squeeze the spot, and all nurses should understand that any septic condition of the nose, or indeed of any part of the face must be regarded seriously. There is danger of the infections spreading to the orbit and so to the cavernous sinus. A rigor, pyrexia associated with headache, and swelling of the eyelids would indicate the serious condition of sinus thrombosis. Cellulitis of the whole face sometimes accompanies nasal furunculosis.

Treatment. The small, solitary furuncle is rarely treated with antibiotics, but with recurrence one of these is given. Sometimes, local treatment of the nose will give relief—for example, frequent hot bathing, or plugging the nostril with ribbon gauze well soaked in hot normal saline. Too strong a salt solution must be avoided as it is liable to damage the surrounding skin and mucous membrane and leave the nose very sore. An analgesic drug, such as aspirin or an aspirin compound, will probably be necessary to relieve pain and enable the patient to sleep at night. Vitamins A, B, C and D should be given to help raise the patient's resistance against infection. Should there be pyrexia, rest in bed is indicated. When the 'pointing' stage of the boil is complete, a light touch with a sterile wound probe will hasten the expulsion of the core and promote drainage, or the boil may be left to discharge itself.

To prevent recurrence, the inside of the nostril may be painted with an antiseptic solution such as gentian violet 1%. The hairs inside the nostril should be kept closely clipped. For persistent recurrence, the use of autogenous vaccine has met with some success. A holiday and attention to the general health are advised.

Cavernous sinus thrombosis

This very serious condition may be an extension of thrombosis of the angular vein, caused by furunculosis of the nose. The septic thrombus travels to the cavernous sinus via the ophthalmic vein. If there is slow occlusion of the sinus, a collateral circulation is set up. The patient is desperately ill.

Signs and symptoms. There are recurrent rigors, the temperature rising to 40.6°C (105°F). Nausea and vomiting frequently occur. Pain in the orbit and side of the head is acute and there is intense progressive oedema of the eyelids. The eyeball is protruded and paralysis of the eye muscles follows, due to the involvement of the cranial nerves in the cavernous sinus. There may be ptosis, squint and alterations in the pupils.

Treatment. The usual nursing for patients with intermittent pyrexia and sweating will be needed. Recovery depends largely upon the early administration of antibiotics, anticoagulants and treatment of the primary infection.

Lupus vulgaris

This is a chronic inflammation, now uncommon, of the skin of the nose and cheeks, caused by invasion by the tubercle bacillus. Occasionally it attacks the trunk and limbs. The first sign is the appearance of one or more tiny reddish or reddish-brown papules, surrounded by an area of hyperaemia. When pressed by glass, the spots have an 'apple jelly' appearance. They gradually enlarge, forming an irregular patch of soft nodules which often ulcerate, crust and heal with scarring. Healing occurs in one part of the affected area, while spread is taking place at another. The ulcers are superficial and scars are yellowish and shrunken. The disease occurs in children and young adults. It is painless, but there is often much destruction of cartilage and bone. Occasionally the nose is destroyed, or carcinoma may develop.

Treatment. General treatment consists of a highly nourishing diet, with additional vitamins. Calciferol is given in large doses for at least a year. Ultraviolet light may be employed. Streptomycin, para-aminosalicylic acid and isonicotinic acid may also be given.

Lupus erythematosus

This disease is differentiated from lupus vulgaris as there are no nodules or ulcers. There are reddish patches covered at times with an adherent scale, and there is a tendency to scarring. When on the nose, the disease often extends on to the cheeks in a butterfly-shaped patch. It is a local manifestation of what is generally a systemic disease.

Treatment. There should be protection of the face from strong sunlight. Systemic steroids are given.

Frostbite

Owing to its exposed position, the nose is one of the first parts of the body to be affected by frostbite. An extremely low atmospheric temperature will cause pain in the extremities of the body until they become frozen. At this stage the skin is white and shining and pain ceases. Because of this the victim of frostbite may be unaware of its occurrence, and prolonged exposure may lead to necrosis of tissue. As thawing of the part takes place, the surface blood vessels dilate once more, and if this is sudden, the pain may be intense. The engorgement is followed by stasis of blood in the capillaries, exudation of serum and the formation of blisters, very similar to the injury caused by burns.

Treatment. The first step in the treatment of frostbite is the *very gradual* restoration of warmth and normal circulation in the part. This is best achieved by keeping the patient in a moderately warm room. Heat must not be applied to the nose, nor must the patient be allowed near the fire. The later treatment of the frostbitten area is similar to that of burns.

An ointment, powder or sterile dressing material impregnated with an antibiotic may be applied. Pain is relieved by analgesia.

Syphilis of the nose

A primary syphilitic chancre on the nose is almost unknown, but secondary syphilis may produce lesions around the alae at the same time as on other parts of the body. Infants suffering from congenital syphilis frequently develop mucous patches which extend into the nasal cavity and cause 'snuffles'. Gummatous destruction of bone tissue may give rise to a depression of the bridge of the nose, known as 'saddle nose'. This usually appears at about one year of age.

Tertiary syphilis may manifest itself as firm, painless nodules or as gummatous ulcers with deep sharp-cut edges, which, when healed, leave soft, smooth, whitish scars, described as 'tissue paper'. These ulcers are very destructive and common sites for them are about the nasal apertures and the lips.

Treatment. The method of treatment of syphilis is the injection of penicillin procaine.

New growths of the nose

Small benign growths such as papillomata (warts) and angiomata (naevi) may occur on the nose and be removed, if desirable, by cautery or diathermy. The most common malignant growth of the nose is carcinoma.

Epithelioma, or squamous-celled carcinoma

The first sign is the formation of small, waxy nodules or warts, which gradually extend or deepen. Ulceration of the centre occurs, with crusting and bleeding. The edge of the ulcer is raised and rolled out. If the growth is allowed to develop, it may penetrate the nose. External irradiation, radium therapy or removal by scalpel or diathermy knife under local anaesthetic are the common methods of treatment. Healing after excision takes several weeks, and if the growth has penetrated to the mucous membrane, plastic surgery may be needed later.

Rodent ulcer — basal-celled carcinoma

This growth arises from cells in the sebaceous glands of the hair follicles or from the basal cells in the epidermis, and most commonly develops on the face. A common site is at the entrance to the nostrils. The growth may be mistaken for a simple inflammatory lesion, and careful examination is necessary. The base of the rodent ulcer is depressed and crusted, and the edge is pearly and slightly raised —

the 'rolled edge'. Rodent ulcers develop slowly and are curable if diagnosed early. They are only locally malignant and do not invade the lymphatic system. The treatment is by irradiation or excision.

Foreign bodies in the nose

A foreign body has been defined as a substance not normally connected with its surroundings. Peas, beans and other small objects are commonly pushed into the nose by children without causing grave emergency. However, since the removal without causing further damage is difficult, such patients should be taken to a doctor or a hospital.

Foreign bodies remaining impacted in the nose give rise to discharge on the affected side, either of blood or pus. If the foreign body is seen to be smooth and rounded, the simplest method of removal is to pass a blunt-pointed director along the floor of the nose, under and behind the object, and then to gently withdraw it. This procedure is only carried out by a nurse if she has undergone supervised training. In this case, the nurse will have a written statement of authorization from her employing authority. Should the object be jagged or firmly impacted, the surgeon must remove it. The nose should be cocainized. Adrenaline may be added to the solution in order to cause shrinkage of the mucous membrane. Sometimes a general anaesthetic is given. Removal of the object is effected with forceps using a nasal speculum under good illumination.

Broken nose, and soft-tissue wounds of the face

In a direct blow on the face, the nose usually takes the main brunt of the force. The weak nasal bones readily yield, and the walls of the sinuses may give way if the violence is great. There is considerable bruising and swelling, and usually haemorrhage from the nose. The first-aid treatment must avoid direct interference — there must be no blowing of the nose, douching or packing. Alternate hot and cold bathing may relieve pain and swelling.

Any wounds of the soft tissue of the face should receive early treatment. All dirt must be removed and debris cleared. Systemic chemotherapy is advisable.

Once the swelling has subsided and clear X-rays have been taken, the surgeon will reduce the fracture. This may be two to three days after the injury.

Epistaxis, or nose bleeding

Bleeding from the nose is one of the most common forms of haemorrhage. It occurs especially in children and the elderly, very rarely in infants. The causes are legion, more often local than general disorders.

Causes. Of the local disorders, the more common are (*a*) injury, and (*b*) superficial ulceration of inflammatory origin.

Among the general disorders, the commonest cause is a raised blood pressure. Blood diseases such as leukaemia, anaemia and haemophilia will also cause frequent epistaxis.

The bleeding in almost every case begins from a point on the septum called Kiesselbach's or Little's area, about 6 mm inside the vestibule. At this spot is a very rich supply of blood vessels, both arteries and veins, whose thin walls readily become eroded.

Apart from the underlying causes and some head injuries, epistaxis is rarely serious. In most instances, it ceases spontaneously in a few minutes.

Treatment. The first-aid treatment consists of pressure. The patient can immediately nip his own nose. Usually the bleeding is from one nostril only, though this is not always apparent at first. At the start the patient should blow his nose to clear loose clots. He should sit on a chair by a table and be given a pad of absorbent wool to hold against the nose. The elbow of the side that is bleeding should rest on the table. The nose can then be pressed against the thumb in an easy and comfortable position. The opposite nostril is free for respiratory purposes and, the head being kept forward, blood is not so liable to trickle down the pharynx.

Only too often, patients have been advised to hold the head back — this causes blood to be swallowed and results in nausea and vomiting, an unnecessary and distressing complication, which leads to further bleeding.

The patient may be given a cork or something similar to bite on. With a cork in the mouth he cannot easily swallow or breathe through his nose or move his palate. This puts the nose at rest and discourages bleeding.

When epistaxis does not spontaneously cease, the nose is packed with ribbon gauze impregnated with liquid paraffin to which has been added iodoform paste. The packing may be left in place for several days if the patient is given antibiotic 'cover', but is usually removed after 24 hours. An application of a 1 in 10 000 solution of venom from Russell's viper usually causes immediate clotting but is only useful if the bleeding point can be seen. Adrenaline solution may temporarily constrict vessels, but as its effect wears off, bleeding is apt to recur.

Morphine is ordered in severe cases for rest and sleep. The nurse should record the pulse rate and blood pressure every half hour, and give an estimate of the blood loss. An intravenous infusion may be needed to maintain the fluid and electrolyte balance. With severe or prolonged epistaxis, a transfusion of packed cells or blood may be required.

In cases of bleeding at intervals, if the bleeding point can be easily seen and dealt with, a cautery may be used to seal the vessel. A swab of cotton wool, soaked in 10% cocaine solution (or 25% cocaine paste) is first applied to the bleeding point. After cauterization, the patient must be warned not to blow his nose for three days.

Very rarely, when epistaxis cannot be arrested by other means, ligation of the external carotid or ethmoidal artery is necessary.

AFFECTIONS OF THE INTERNAL NOSE

Diseases of the nasal septum

Deviation of the septum

The septum is seldom a simple straight partition dividing the cavity. The deviation may be congenital or it may be due to injury. Frequently a blow or fall at an early age, unnoticed at the time or quickly forgotten, may cause bending of the cartilage which then ossifies crookedly. The perpendicular plate of the ethmoid bone is often so markedly to one side that it almost touches the middle turbinate and interferes with the ventilation and drainage of the sinuses. Cartilaginous deviation is in the interior portion of the nose and is usually obvious on sight. It often involves the upper part of the quadrilateral cartilage. With severe injury the cartilage may be destroyed or project into the opposite nostril. Injuries in later life, especially if repeated as in boxing, may cause such great irregularity that both sides of the nose become obstructed.

Bony or cartilaginous outgrowths, called 'spurs', may occur on the septum, but these seldom give rise to symptoms of nasal obstruction. When the septum is deflected very much to one side, a large cavity is left in the opposite nostril, and the inferior turbinate then enlarges (see Fig. 11.1), which makes correction more complicated.

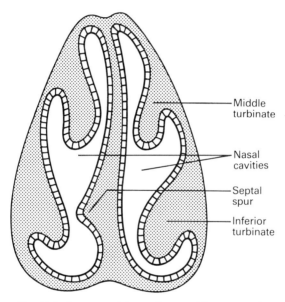

Fig. 11.1. *Deviation of the nasal septum (diagrammatic).*

When deviation of the septum is sufficient to cause nasal obstruction on either side, the mucous membrane becomes congested and oedematous. The openings from the sinuses become blocked, and, owing to stagnation of the secretion and consequent infection, the patients are particularly liable to colds and to sinusitis. Correction of the deformity is by surgery (see Submucous Resection of the Septum, p. 95), but not as a rule under 18 years of age, lest the nasal bridge should collapse for lack of the support normally provided by the septum.

Haematoma of the septum

This is a collection of blood between the layers of the septum, usually due to injury. There may be external bruising and tenderness over the bridge of the nose, but the chief symptom is partial or complete nasal obstruction on both sides of the nose. The condition is diagnosed by inspection and palpation, or a diagnostic puncture may be made.

Treatment. A haematoma often becomes infected, in which case necrosis of cartilage will follow. Incision near the floor of the nose, on both sides of the septum if necessary, is therefore advisable. The incision is made with a narrow-bladed knife under local anaesthesia, the blood clot is evacuated and a small drain of ribbon gauze is inserted.

Abscess of the septum

The usual cause of abscess of the septum is secondary infection of a haematoma, but abscesses occasionally follow an acute infection such as measles or typhoid fever, or are due to upward spread from a decayed incisor tooth root. The signs of suppuration are pyrexia, swelling and throbbing pain. The nose is slightly swollen and the skin is red and shining especially over the bridge and tip.

Treatment. As soon as fluctuation is apparent, there should be incision of the abscess, as described for haematoma. Antibiotic or sulphonamide powder may be dusted into the abscess cavity, and an antibiotic given systematically. It may be necessary to reinsert ribbon gauze daily for a few days, to keep the free drainage. A small roll of sterile gauze may be fastened under the nose to absorb drainage, and the patient's upper lip should be protected by ointment.

Complications. The abscess usually takes about a week to heal, leaving no after-effects, but occasionally perforation of the septum occurs, and necrosis is comparatively common. Necrosis leads to collapse of the nasal apex.

Perforation of the septum

This may follow various ulcerating diseases affecting the nose, or suppuration, injury, and particularly, inveterate nose-picking. The perforation may be quite symptomless, or a whistling sound may be present on either inspiration or expiration.

Treatment. The treatment is that of the disease. Plastic repair may be performed.

INFLAMMATORY CONDITIONS OF THE NOSE

Acute catarrhal rhinitis or coryza

These are synonymous terms applied to the inflammation of the mucous membrane of the nose known as the 'common cold' which has already been discussed to some extent in Chapter 1. There is irritation of the mucous membrane producing sneezing, with dilatation of the mucus-secreting glands (goblet cells) and of blood vessels. At first the discharge consists of clear mucus, and after 12–24 hours, the nose becomes obstructed by the swollen mucous membrane. The eyes often water as the inflammation spreads up the lacrimal duct, and there is headache and malaise. These symptoms are due to many types of virus. Secondary bacterial infection commonly leads to further symptoms:

1. Purulent rhinitis, the nasal discharge becoming purulent and thick.
2. Sinusitis.
3. Laryngitis and cough, due to post-nasal discharge.

The acute stage of a cold lasts from two days to one week, after which the symptoms subside and the nasal mucous membrane returns to normal in 1–3 weeks. The temperature rarely rises above 37°C (99°F).

Acute rhinitis must be closely observed whenever it occurs during an epidemic. In *scarlet fever*, the temperature rises sharply to about 39°C (102°F) and there is marked sore throat and backache. A rash appears on the second day of the illness. In *measles*, Koplik's spots appear inside the cheeks on the second day. On the third day the temperature rises to about 39.5°C (103°F) and on the fourth day the rash appears. With *influenza*, there is more general malaise with aching of the limbs, and fewer nasal symptoms.

The principles to be followed are:

1. Isolation of the patient.
2. Relief of symptoms.
3. Prevention of secondary infection.

Treatment of acute rhinitis. At the onset of a cold, it is in the patient's own interest and that of others that he should go to bed. Aspirin and copious fluids, preferably hot, will relieve the headache and sore throat.

After a day or two, symptoms subside and treatment may be reduced. The nose must be kept clear of discharge and crusts, and all coughs and sneezes guarded by a handkerchief. The correct use and treatment of handkerchiefs has already been mentioned. It is advisable to smear the upper lip and around the vestibule of the nose with a mild ointment to prevent cracks.

Herpes simplex

Herpes simplex or 'cold sores', frequently appear around the mouth following a cold. The predisposing cause is a virus which resides in the skin of certain individuals whose tendency to herpes is aggravated by any condition causing irritation. Vesicles occur on the lips and cause constant 'tickling' discomfort. After about 24 hours the vesicles rupture and crusts are formed. If left alone, healing rapidly takes place. But if the patient succumbs to the great temptation to pick off irritating crusts this leads to bleeding areas and delay in recovery.

Treatment. Since herpes simplex is so common, the remedies advocated are legion. Most sufferers have their favourite applications. A quickly drying ointment with a basis of zinc oxide or collodion, applied to the lip at the onset of discomfort may avert or limit the outbreak, and a spirituous application to the ulcer will relieve pain and hasten the healing.

Chronic rhinitis

Recurrent attacks of acute rhinitis, due to some underlying cause which prevents free drainage of the nose, lead to permanent changes in the nasal mucosa, and then the condition becomes chronic. Such causes are, commonly, disease of the paranasal sinuses, adenoids, or deviation of the nasal septum, and less commonly, occupation in a dusty atmosphere. Sometimes, however, no cause is found.

There are several types of chronic rhinitis.

Chronic hypertrophic rhinitis

In this type of chronic rhinitis the mucous membrane, especially over the posterior part of the inferior turbinate process, is thick and oedematous. There is an abnormal secretion of thin sticky mucus. The patient cannot breathe through the nose, and mouth breathing leads frequently to pharyngitis and laryngitis. There is constant headache and lassitude. When treated with vasoconstrictors, the mucous membrane fails to shrink completely, as there is dilatation and thickening of the blood vessels, enlargement of the mucous glands and interstitial fibrosis. The treatment consists of removing the cause; sinusitis may be treated, deviation of the septum corrected. The patient is advised to avoid smoking and alcohol. Cauterization may be employed to contract the thickened mucosa.

Chronic atrophic rhinitis

This is a disappearing disease. It becomes evident at puberty, and the sufferers are often women who have been undernourished in the past. Its cause is probably connected with some neglected infection. There is drying, shrinking and fibrosis of the mucous membrane, followed by atrophy of the turbinate bones, so that the nasal fossae appear particularly spacious, and the nasopharynx can easily be seen. The mucosa is pale. The patient complains of constant crust-formation in the nose. The crusts are greenish and may become very offensive, when the condition is known as ozoena. The foul odour (which is often unnoticed by the patient herself, since the sense of smell is lost), is thought to be due to the invasion of bacilli, which, however, do not cause the atrophy.

Treatment. The nostrils must be kept as clean as possible. Saline irrigations are used, and once daily this may be followed by spraying the nose with oestrogen in oil. The oestrogen may be gradually reduced to weekly or fortnightly treatment, or a watery solution of glucose and glycerine may be used.

Allergic rhinitis — hay fever

Allergy of the respiratory mucous membrane is usually due to irritation from pollen (especially grasses, hence its common title), household or occupational dust, cosmetics containing orris root, or moulds. The condition may be complicated by food allergy.

The symptoms are irritation in the anterior nares, violent sneezing, watery nasal discharge, and often streaming eyes. The nose is obstructed, the mucous membrane typically being pale and oedematous, although it occasionally appears normal or slightly red. When a specimen of the nasal discharge is stained and examined in the laboratory, eosinophils (acid-staining leucocytes) are found to be present in large numbers. Other manifestations of allergy, such as asthma or urticaria, may point to a diagnosis.

Skin tests are made by scratch or intradermal injection to discover the particular sensitivity of individual patients, such substances being used as the extracts of foodstuffs, pollens, and the dandruff of animals. When tests have shown the origin of the allergy, diluted extract of the offending material is injected subcutaneously in order to desensitize the patient. Slowly increasing doses at weekly intervals are given early in the year. If too big a dose is given, intense hay-fever symptoms and severe urticaria occur. These are relieved by antihistamine tablets. Pure 'hay fever' is caused only by pollen. Should the cause of the allergy be undetected, injections of mixed proteins may be tried.

Treatment. Antihistamic drugs such as promethazine hydrochloride (Phenergan), phenindamine tartrate (Thephorin) and chlorpheniramine maleate (Piriton) provide great relief when given by mouth, three times daily. Otherwise little can be done for the patient at the time of the attack, which may last intermittently for several days, except to relieve the exhaustion caused by the violent sneezing. The sufferer should avoid over-heating — either by a fire or too warm bedclothes, as this intensifies the symptoms.

The electric cautery or diathermy may be applied to the inferior turbinate processes if there is hypertrophy in the obstinate, chronic, non-seasonal case, but unless there is marked deformity, operation should be avoided.

MISCELLANEOUS CONDITIONS OF THE NOSE

Nasal polypi

These are benign overgrowths of fibrovascular tissue which develop from the oedematous mucous membrane caused by nasal allergy or long-standing infection. The polypi are large greyish masses, usually multiple, and have the appearance of a bunch of grapes. They are usually pedunculated and project into the nose, sometimes appearing at the anterior nares. Polypi most often arise in the ethmoid sinuses, sometimes from the middle turbinates, or from the antra, and may cause marked obstruction, a nasal voice and headaches.

They may block the posterior nares, when they are called choanal polypi. Occasionally the surface of polypi may become ulcerated or haemorrhagic, causing purulent discharge or epistaxis, respectively.

Treatment. Occasionally a polypus is blown out of the nose, or disappears, but surgical removal with a snare is usually required. Unless the underlying cause can be removed, polypi will recur.

Tuberculosis of the nasal cavity

Lupus vulgaris (previously discussed) may spread from the skin around the vestibule into the nasal cavity. It causes severe ulceration and destruction of the soft parts of the nose. There is a subacute variety which manifests itself as flat, pale vegetations, which break down into ulcers. There is usually no ozoena, and the condition may be confined to the nasal cavity for a long time.

Treatment. Blood tests are made to exclude syphilis, and microscopic examination of a small portion of mucous membrane may be made to confirm the diagnosis. A strict regimen for the general treatment of tuberculosis is necessary until the disease is under control. The warty growths may be coagulated by diathermy, or cautery, or application of chromic acid, after crusts have been removed by a mild alkaline solution. Patients must be encouraged to keep up out-patient attendance long after apparent cure.

Nasal diphtheria — membranous rhinitis

There are times when the *Corynebacterium diphtheriae* will attack the nose as a primary infection without affecting the larynx. The patient is not as a rule acutely ill. There is nasal obstruction and a sudden, unilateral blood-stained discharge, and on examination, a greyish-white membrane can sometimes be seen on the inferior turbinate bone and adjacent parts. When the membrane is removed, a bleeding area is left.

Treatment. As soon as the disease is recognized, without waiting for laboratory tests, the patient is isolated, given antitoxin, and arrangements are made for him to be removed to an infectious-diseases unit.

Choanal atresia

In this rare condition, which may be congenital or acquired, the posterior nares are blocked by membrane or bone. If acquired, it is due to injury or to severe infection, such as diphtheria or tuberculosis, followed by scarring. The chief symptom of atresia is the absence of breathing in the affected side. When the condition is congenital and bilateral, it is noticed from birth that the child is unable to breathe and suck at the same time. Examination reveals the blockage. Surgical removal of the obstructing membrane or bone is required. It can be a matter of great urgency in the newborn child if the condition is bilateral, owing to difficulty with breathing and feeding.

12 Diseases of the paranasal sinuses

Acute maxillary sinusitis

When considering this condition, it is as well to remember that in a young child the second dentition in the maxillary bones develops at a short distance below the orbits. The descent of the teeth is due to the laying down of new bone. Some air spaces are present in the bone at birth, and these increase in size, eventually forming the large maxillary air sinuses or antra. At about nine years of age the floors of the maxillary sinuses are at the same level as the floor of the nose. The sinuses are fully formed when the third molars (wisdom teeth) are cut — at about the twenty-fifth year. They then extend from the second premolar to the third molar teeth, upwards to the floors of the orbits, and sideways to the wall of the nose at the level of the inferior turbinate (see Fig. 1.1, p. 4). Above this, in the wall of the middle meatus, is the ostium into the nose from each sinus. A small accessory opening is often found in front of and below the ostia. A division of the inferior orbital nerve crosses the roof of each maxillary sinus and a division of the superior alveolar nerve lies in the floor of each sinus.

Symptoms. Acute infection of a maxillary sinus is usually a sequel to acute rhinitis due to spread by continuity through the maxillary ostium or the accessory opening, or may result from infection of a tooth root in the floor of the sinus. The chief predisposing factor is a blocked middle meatus. Pain and tenderness occur in the cheek, in the teeth on the affected side, and over the eye. The last symptom may imply involvement of the frontal sinus.

Treatment. The initial treatment is that of an ordinary cold. Pain may be relieved by analgesics, and by heat in the form of either a steam inhalation or an external application. The attack often disappears spontaneously, but should the symptoms be severe, an antibiotic is often given. Should pain and discharge continue, then a trocar and cannula can be passed into the nose, and the wall between the sinus and the nose can be punctured (antrum, or proof puncture), and the sinuses irrigated. Occasionally a permanent opening in the wall of the inferior meatus is needed (intranasal antrostomy).

With a subacute infection, suction displacement therapy with ephedrine or an antibiotic solution may cure the condition.

Chronic maxillary sinusitis

Signs. Recurrent attacks of acute sinusitis, or an acute attack which fails to resolve will become a chronic condition. There is persistent nasal and post-nasal discharge, but no fever. On examination, pus can be seen in the middle meatus and on the back wall of the pharynx. The diagnosis is confirmed by transillumination and X-ray appearances.

Treatment. Every factor that might hinder free drainage of the sinus should receive attention. Polypi should be removed, a deviated septum should be corrected. These measures may be sufficient, but if necessary repeated antrum irrigation should be performed. Operations should be undertaken only when the lining membrane of the antrum is irreversibly altered, i.e. shows itself incapable of return to the normal state. Caldwell–Luc's operation is a radical removal of the thickened mucous membrane. This operation is an alternative to the intranasal antrostomy in many centres.

Frontal sinusitis

Since the frontal sinuses are late in developing, inflammation of them is not found under six years of age.

Some inflammation of the frontal sinuses may occur with maxillary sinusitis and may persist as chronic frontal sinusitis.

Symptoms. The patient complains of heaviness and tenderness over the eyes and of an inability to concentrate. Frontal headache is usual. As a rule it is absent on rising, comes on during the morning, reaching its maximum at noon, and has gone by tea time. If the pain does not lessen at night, the conclusion is that natural drainage of the sinus is absent. There is often copious discharge. The discharge is most marked on rising, and, on examination, pus can be seen to cover the thickened mucous membrane in the middle meatus of the nose. The frontal sinus is opaque in a radiograph.

Nasal polypi are sometimes present. Obstruction of the naso-frontal duct may give rise to a mucocele—a cyst in the sinus containing mucus. This must be completely removed as it may become infected, or increase in size and erode the orbit.

Treatment. All patients with acute frontal sinusitis should be in bed. Pain may be relieved by analgesics, and by heat in the form of either a steam inhalation or an external application. If these measures do not relieve the patient's distress, then a small burr-hole is made into the floor of the frontal sinus and a drainage tube is inserted.

Ethmoidal sinusitis

A patient who suffers from maxillary or frontal sinusitis has always an associated inflammation of the ethmoid sinuses. In a child, the ethmoid sinusitis may be the presenting disease in an acute case.

Symptoms. These are largely obscured by those of the maxillary or frontal sinusitis.

Treatment. This is included in that of the larger affected sinus and is usually conservative. In infants, however, where the infection presents as swelling, incision and drainage may be needed.

Sphenoidal sinusitis

Inflammation of the sphenoid sinus is very uncommon but as a rule responds quickly to simple treatment.

Symptoms. The headache in this condition differentiates it from the other forms of sinus infections with which it is associated. There is occipital pain, which may spread over the mastoid process, and there may be pain at the back of the eye. Other symptoms of acute sphenoid sinusitis are stiffness of the neck muscles; vague unsteadiness, which may be continuous or intermittent, and is increased on turning the head; sleeplessness due chiefly to periodic discharge from the sinus into the throat; dryness at the back of the nose; and a persistent, tickling, throaty cough. The discharge is thick and can be seen coming from behind the palate.

If chronic sphenoid sinusitis supervenes, the headache becomes continuous, and is increased on exercise, smoking or drinking alcohol. Toxaemia may cause mental depression and inability to concentrate. Ocular symptoms such as exophthalmos and visual disturbances occur late. A dry throat is typical.

Complications. The complications of severe untreated acute sphenoid sinusitis are likely to be serious. That most to be feared is cavernous sinus thrombosis. Partial or complete blindness may develop.

Treatment. The acute case is treated by antibiotics. Vary rarely is anything further needed. The chronic case may be treated by removing the anteroinferior sinus wall. To achieve this, part of the septum may need resection.

Paranasal tumours

New growths of the paranasal sinuses are uncommon, but are more often malignant than benign. They are usually carcinomata arising from the ethmoid or the maxillary antrum. The growth may extend into the nose (causing unilateral obstruction, discharge and epistaxis), into the orbit (displacing the eye), downwards into the hard palate, or outwards causing swelling of the cheek. Pain is characteristic.

The treatment consists of irradiation followed by wide removal of involved bone.

13 Surgical operations on the nose and paranasal sinuses

Preparation of the patient

The general preparation of a patient for a nasal operation is as for any other surgical operation. The patient's heart, lungs and urine are examined. X-rays of the sinuses will be taken, and bacteriological examinations made of nose and throat swabs. The operation is postponed if the patient is suffering from an acute infection — for example, coryza, tonsillitis or acute sinusitis. Starvation increases the tendency to vomiting and most patients can be given a normal, but easily digested diet, up to six hours before operation (unless other directions are given). A patient is well advised to refrain from smoking for 24 hours before operation.

The local preparation consists of cleaning the vestibule of the nose, the mouth and the upper lip. Some surgeons prefer the lip shaved. If not, any moustache must be washed carefully and the lip rendered as clean as possible. Immediately before the operation, the patient is given a mouthwash. Patients will usually be ordered a preoperative sedative.

Nasal operations are performed under local or general anaesthesia. For both types, the nose is sprayed and gauze-packed with 10% cocaine solution, or it is painted with 25% cocaine paste, or postural instillation of cocaine may be adopted. In the last case the cocaine solution is instilled into the nose with the patient in various positions — right lateral, knee-elbow and left lateral positions for five minutes each. The nurse should explain to the patient the reasons for this exercise.

Submucous resection of the septum

The patient is made comfortable, either sitting up or lying on the operating table, with his head and shoulders slightly raised on a pillow. If local anaesthetic is used his eyes are bandaged or covered with a sterile towel which is placed under his head. He is reassured and encouraged to relax with his hands lying flat and limp at his sides. The sterile towels are then secured to cover his body completely from toes to chin and his head with the exception of the area to be operated upon. The nasal packs are withdrawn and the skin of the nose and upper lip are mopped with a skin-sterilizing agent.

To supplement the preoperative cocainization, the surgeon may inject 1 in 1000 Nupercaine solution or Xylocaine into the mucous membrane on each side of the septum. He makes an incision with a small sharp-pointed knife on one side of the septum. The mucous membrane is then lifted with a flat-sided elevator from the cartilage and bone on that side. Next, the septal cartilage is incised and the mucous membrane elevated on the other side, great care being taken to avoid perforating this layer of mucous membrane. The surgeon then removes a portion of the cartilage and bone. Any bony spurs are removed with a sharp elevator or a fish-tail gouge and mallet. When the airway is perfectly clear, the septal flaps of mucous membrane are replaced to meet. It is usual to pack each nostril in order to keep the two layers of membrane together and prevent a blood clot forming between them. The packing may be done with ribbon gauze soaked in liquid paraffin, or with rubber finger-stalls stuffed with gauze and lubricated with petroleum jelly, or some form of nasal splint. Stitching is usually not required. It is customary to place a wool filament gauze bolster under the external nares and to secure it with adhesive (see Fig. 13.1).

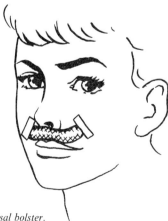

Fig. 13.1. *Nasal bolster.*

After-treatment. The patient must not on any account blow his nose, for fear of causing bleeding and haematoma. Sterile gauze swabs are provided for mopping any blood that oozes from the nostrils. The nurse should find out from the surgeon when the nasal packs, if any, are to be removed. (In special cases they may be left 24 or even 48 hours.) The patient should lie quietly for half an hour after removal of the pack, to prevent haemorrhage.

Four-hourly steam inhalations, usually with tincture of benzoin, are given as routine treatment, preceded by drops of mild silver protein and ephedrine drops. The patient will be discharged from hospital 7–10 days after the operation, and it is inadvisable for him to return to work within a further two weeks. He should also be advised that violent exercise should be avoided for the first month following the operation. Should epistaxis occur, he should report to the hospital, as great care must be taken to prevent haematoma of the septum.

The patient should be taught the method of compressing the septum to arrest epistaxis before he is discharged from the ward. He should be warned that relief from nasal obstruction will not be immediate and is delayed for some weeks, till healing has been completed.

Removal of nasal polypi

This operation may be performed in the out-patients' department, and is often combined with other operations on the nasal sinuses. If the patient has many polypi, or if sinus infection is present, he is admitted to the ward, and after operation is kept in bed for two or three days and treated with menthol or friar's balsam inhalations.

To remove the polypi, the nose is cocainized. A wire snare is passed round the base of each lobule of polypus which is avulsed. Before sterilizing the snare, the nurse should ensure that the wire is unbroken and the loop is straight. Small polypi may be removed with Luc's forceps. If there is much bleeding, the nose is packed, but usually a little cotton wool to mop up any drops of blood is sufficient.

Cauterization of the nose

A galvanocautery handle and points and a nasal speculum are

required. The cautery is usually heated by a transformer from the mains. When the nose has been anaesthetized, the current is turned on until the cautery point warms to a bright red. It is then applied to the tissues round the bleeding point. The cautery is removed from the nose before the current is turned off and the cautery point is cleaned by passing the current through it until all secretions are burned away. It is then detached from the handle and put away. After cauterization, the patient is given some ointment to apply daily to the nostril until the area is healed.

Proof puncture of the maxillary sinus (intranasal antrotomy or antral puncture)

The patient is prepared by having the inferior meatus of the affected side cocainized. A Lichtwitz trocar and cannula is inserted into the inferior meatus and the wall of the sinus is pierced at a point about 2.5 cm from the anterior end of the turbinate process (see Fig. 13.2). The trocar is then withdrawn leaving the cannula in position. A 10 ml syringe which contains 3 or 4 ml of normal saline is fitted to the Lichtwitz cannula. The plunger of the syringe is withdrawn to aspirate the fluid contents of the cavity. If nothing is obtained, the saline is injected and withdrawn from the sinus. Pus may be

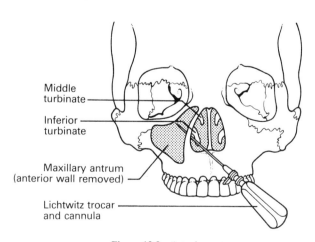

Middle turbinate

Inferior turbinate

Maxillary antrum (anterior wall removed)

Lichtwitz trocar and cannula

Figure 13.2. *Antral puncture.*

obtained, of which a specimen is sent to the pathological laboratory for examination. If return of the fluid does not follow the injection of saline, it is probable that the sinus is full of polypoid tissue, or that the needle has penetrated too far. If the proof puncture is positive, and purulent fluid is returned, a Higginson's syringe can be attached to the cannula and the sinus washed out. The Higginson's syringe must be quite full of fluid before it is attached. The fluid passes through the natural ostium of the sinus, into the nose, and then out into a receiver held under the patient's chin.

After irrigation, a small quantity of 0.5% ephedrine in normal saline, or an appropriate antibiotic in solution, is sometimes injected into the cavity, through the cannula.

As a rule, the patient is kept at rest for half an hour following the operation, and may then go home. A little oozing of blood-stained serum is to be expected for two or three days.

Sometimes the surgeon decides on a daily antral washout for a week or so. To avoid repeated puncture, a fine polythene tube may be passed through the cannula into the antrum and left in position on withdrawing the cannula (see Fig. 13.3). The tube is fastened to the nose and forehead with strapping, and through it irrigation or the instillation of an antibiotic solution can easily be carried out. This method is used especially for children, thus avoiding repeated general anaesthetics.

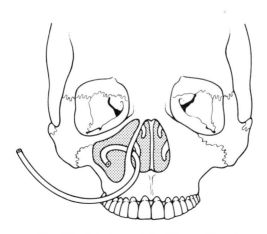

Fig. 13.3. *Polythene tube in right maxillary sinus.*

Intranasal antrostomy (antral window)

This operation establishes a temporary or permanent opening into the maxillary sinus to permit repeated lavage when medical treatment and proof puncture have failed to cure subacute sinusitis. The anterior end of the inferior turbinate bone is dislocated upwards, or, if necessary, is removed with punch forceps, and an opening through the wall of the sinus is made with a trephine or other perforating instrument. The opening is made as low and as far forward as possible. It is enlarged with biting forceps and an antrum chisel. Pus usually wells out of the sinus at this stage. The cavity is washed out and the ephedrine or antibiotic solution injected as for simple antral puncture (above).

Radical antrostomy (Caldwell–Luc's operation)

When the mucous membrane is grossly infected, or when polypi are present in the maxillary sinus, the whole lining must be removed. The approach to the antrum is under the upper lip, in the canine fossa. No preoperative packing is required, but the nose is usually cocainized before the operation.

Sometimes the operation is performed under general anaesthesia given by the intratracheal route. The post-nasal space and the pharynx can then be packed to prevent blood and secretions from entering the trachea.

If general anaesthesia is required, the patient is usually given a preoperative hypodermic injection of atropine sulphate 0.6 mg. Before a local anaesthetic, papaveretum (Omnopon) 30–40 mg is given.

When the patient is on the operation table, either the local or the general anaesthetic is supplemented by cinchocaine hydrochloride (Nupercaine) 0.5 or 1% with adrenaline 1 in 1000 in the proportion of 0.3 ml of adrenaline in 30 ml. This, the anaesthetist injects into the area of the incision, above the canine and the first and second molar teeth. If the patient is unconscious, the mouth may be lightly packed with gauze. The upper lip being well retracted, the surgeon makes his incision, and then, with dental drill or hammer and gouge, makes the opening into the antrum. If much bleeding occurs, 1 ml of adrenaline solution is applied on a swab into the cavity. The opening is enlarged with nibbling forceps until the inside of the sinus is visible. Suction apparatus is essential so that the field of operation can be kept clear of blood and purulent fluid. The antral cavity is cleared of diseased mucous membrane and a new opening into the nose is made beneath the inferior turbinate.

A section of the mucous membrane is usually sent to the pathological laboratory for examination. Usually the sinus is left unpacked. A certain amount of oozing of blood and serum is expected for two or three days, and when the opening is no longer required it soon heals. Some surgeons close or partly close the mouth wound with three or four interrupted catgut sutures, which do not need removal, or with wire sutures, which are removed on the fourth day.

Complications. In the case of severe postoperative bleeding, the antrum is irrigated with saline solution at 44°C (110°F), and the nose may need packing. When it is certain that the bleeding has ceased, the packing is removed by the house surgeon or ward sister.

Patients who are bleeding or restless are given morphine 16 mg. Also, an aspirin mixture may be given to relieve headache. After operation some patients complain of neuralgia or anaesthesia of the face for a few days, but this is temporary only and they should be reassured on this point. Frequently swelling of the face occurs and this may be treated by the application of external heat. It usually disappears in four or five days.

Sometimes the eyes become black and swollen. The swelling will subside within 1–2 days.

A more lasting complication is fistula into the mouth. This may be due to the previous removal of a tooth which has caused suppuration and left a patent tooth socket. The treatment is plastic repair.

After-treatment. After all operations on the nose and sinuses strict attention to the mouth toilet is essential. Routine syringing of the antrum is not now commonly practised, but is occasionally ordered if marked sepsis exists. Menthol inhalations and nasal drops may be given 4-hourly. Dentures may be reworn as soon as the patient finds them comfortable. The antrostomy opening into the nose contracts, but does not close completely.

An operation similar to the Caldwell–Luc operation is performed to remove a tumour of the antrum. A routine 'cover' with a sulphonamide or antibiotic is usually ordered by the surgeon for four or five days.

Partial ethmoidectomy

Intranasal operation

This is a simple procedure, frequently combined with other operations on the nose such as antrostomy or the removal of polypi. Under local anaesthesia, the diseased ethmoid cells are scraped out by means of a curette and punch forceps.

External operation

Before operation the eyebrow and skin area are carefully cleaned. A curved incision is made between the bridge of the nose and the eye. Before commencing the operation, the nose is cocainized on the side to be operated on, and both eyes are smeared with sterile petroleum jelly, to prevent blood running into them.

After making the incision, the surgeon divides the structures down to the periosteum, which is retracted. The ethmoid cells are curetted, and drainage is provided into the nose. The external wound is then closed with silkworm gut or silver wire sutures. A small drainage tube is inserted for 24 hours.

An eye pad is bandaged firmly over the eye. If there is swelling or if a tube has been used, a fresh dressing is applied for another 12 or 24 hours. The wound is then left uncovered and the patient is allowed out of bed. Stitches are removed after four days. Should the eye be infected, 10% sulphacetamide or appropriate antibiotic drops may be instilled four times daily.

Operations on the frontal sinus

External operations

The X-rays of the frontal sinuses will indicate their exact size and position, and are therefore of great assistance in these operations.

The trephine operation

This is performed for acute frontal sinusitis. The incision is made between the bridge of the nose and the eye and the tissues are divided down to the bone. In order to avoid penetrating the cancellous bone of the orbital ridge, which might result in osteomyelitis, the entry is made through the compact bone forming the floor of the sinus. The opening is made large enough for a 'portex' tube, 8 mm in diameter, to be inserted. 'Portex' tubing is made of a plastic material, is very smooth and is resistant to pressure. As a rule, the pus drains through this under pressure. The tube is stitched to the skin. The sinus is irrigated through the tube and the fluid passes into the nose when the frontonasal duct reopens.

For chronic frontal sinusitis, there are various operations in practice.

Howarth's operation

The floor of the frontal sinus and part of the anterior ethmoid wall are removed, forming a new channel into the nose.

Negus's operation

This is similar, but the new channel into the nose is lined with a Thiersch graft, to prevent adhesions and the narrowing of the opening by scar tissue.

Before all these operations, the preparation of the patient is similar to that described for external ethmoidectomy. The patient is most often given a general anaesthetic.

When the frontal sinus has been opened, the frontonasal duct is widened and a plastic tube inserted. The latter is brought out through the nostril and left in place for many weeks, according to the directions of the surgeon. It is important that the tube be left until fibrosis has ended. The external wound is closed with silkworm gut or silver wire sutures.

The dressing of the wound is similar to that for ethmoidectomy.

Obliteration of the frontal sinus

Since this operation causes considerable deformity of the upper face, it is rarely performed except in an emergency or for osteomyelitis of the frontal bone. The operation involves the removal of the orbital ridge and the entire outer wall of the sinus.

The osteoplastic operation

This has largely replaced the obliteration operation. An incision is made within the hairline after shaving the vault, and the anterior walls of the frontal sinuses are turned forwards, attached to the scalp. The diseased lining and bone are removed, the ethmoids opened from above and the anterior wall of the sinuses replaced.

Operations for new growth of maxillary antrum

Radiotherapy may precede or *follow* surgical treatment, according to the decision of the surgeon and the radiotherapist in the light of the particular circumstances in each case.

1. If the growth is small and of easy access, excision by the sublabial route (Caldwell–Luc's operation) is carried out.
2. Following external irradiation, the nasal fossa and the maxillary sinus are exposed by removal of the bony walls, including the upper alveolus and hard palate. The growth is coagulated by diathermy and the debris removed. The cavity may be skin-grafted and packed. A bag of gauze, containing strips soaked in iodoform, may be used. This is removed after about a week. A denture carrying an obturator to fill the defect is then inserted to prevent the soft tissues from contracting. If the palate is not involved, an attempt is made to preserve as much as possible in order to facilitate feeding and speech.
3. If the skin of the cheek or the deeper regions of the nose are affected, an external operation (lateral rhinotomy) is performed. This requires subsequent plastic repair.

Trans-sphenoidal hypophysectomy

The removal of the hypophysis (pituitary gland) is an operation performed by ear, nose and throat surgeons. The great majority of hypophysectomies are for uncontrolled breast cancer, particularly when painful bony metastases are present, but the operation can also be used for other diseases. As far as breast cancer is concerned, it is not possible at present to decide in advance which growths are hormone-dependent. About one-third of the patients have a remarkable relief from pain, usually lasting months; in another one-third painful bony metastases and ulcerating skin deposits disappear. In the latter group, the remission may last three or four years.

In trans-sphenoidal hypophysectomy, access is obtained via an external ethmoidectomy, or via the nose or by a combination of these routes. Excellent exposure is obtained without the risks of a major intracranial procedure or of optic nerve injury.

Pre-operative management. The patient is admitted a few days before the operation, and a series of investigations are undertaken:

1. Haemoglobin and blood count.
2. Blood grouping and cross-matching.
3. Blood sugar, blood urea and serum electrolytes.
4. X-rays of chest, skull and sinuses. These should be checked carefully for evidence of metastases, which might affect the type of incision.

Prophylactic antibiotics are commenced. A sulphonamide such as sulphadiazine 1 g 6-hourly may also be used. To combat the hormonal disturbance occasioned by the removal of the pituitary gland, cortisone therapy is begun. Hydrocortisone 100 mg can be given intramuscularly the night before operation and repeated during the morning before operation. If hypophysectomy is undertaken for intractable pain, the patient may be having a considerable amount of analgesia. This should be continued prior to surgery.

The patient should be given an explanation of the various investigations that are being carried out and she should understand the nature of the operation. Close relatives should also be told what is being undertaken and the expected result.

A muscle graft will be needed to pack the pituitary fossa, and for this purpose the right thigh is shaved and the skin cleansed with an antiseptic solution.

The anaesthetist usually sees the patient the day before operation, and prescribes a suitable premedication to be given one to one and a half hours before surgery. A hypnotic will be given to insure a good night's sleep prior to the operation.

At operation, a blood transfusion may be commenced, and a further dose of hydrocortisone may be given. Muscle taken from the thigh is packed into the pituitary fossa with ribbon gauze soaked in liquid paraffin. The pack is brought out through the nose. Raytex ribbon gauze is used to distinguish it from the nasal packs. The wound is sutured. If the external ethmoidal approach is used, an eye pad and bandage may be applied on the affected side. If the nasal approach is made, a nasal splint is applied externally. This is made of gauze soaked in collodion. Both nostrils are packed with ribbon gauze. There is usually a moderate amount of bleeding.

Postoperative management. Usually a general anaesthetic has been given and the patient is nursed flat on her side. The intravenous infusion is continued to maintain fluid and electrolyte balance; a blood transfusion may also have been required. The nurse should observe the patient carefully, particularly noting the general condition, colour, and nature of the respirations. The pulse rate and blood pressure should be taken and recorded at half-hourly intervals for the first few hours. If the systolic pressure falls below 100 mmHg, 100 mg of hydrocortisone may be ordered and given intramuscularly. The patient usually continues to have hydrocortisone 6-hourly until she is able to take drugs orally. Then, prednisolone 50 mg 6-hourly may be ordered instead. The antibiotics and sulphonamide are continued up to 12 days after operation. Analgesics are given as ordered and as required. An aspirin mixture given 4-hourly is found to be very useful and is usually sufficient to control any discomfort after the first 48 hours. A fluid balance chart should be maintained. There may be signs of diabetes insipidus but this can be controlled by intramuscular pitressin.

On the first day the eye pad is removed and the eyes are then bathed with warmed normal saline, 4-hourly. The nasal packs are removed. Once the patient is able to take sufficient fluid orally, the infusion may be discontinued. The patient should be nursed with her head raised on two pillows. She can lie on alternate sides or her back to relieve pressure areas. She may eat and drink whatever she can enjoy. The eyebrow incision sutures are removed on about the fourth day, the nasal sutures at the end of the first week and the thigh sutures about the tenth day. The pituitary pack is removed after the ninth postoperative day. If there is no leak of cerebrospinal fluid, the patient begins to sit out of bed and gradually to walk about in the ward. Thyroid replacement is needed and a small dose of thyroxine, taken orally, is commenced. The dose of prednisolone is gradually reduced. Antibiotics should be discontinued.

Before discharge from hospital the patient should understand the importance of taking the drugs she has been prescribed and particularly the need to increase the dose of prednisolone if she is under stress. She must therefore remain under the close supervision of her doctor or the hospital.

Care of patients who have had a general anaesthetic for operations on the nose and throat

In all cases of nose and throat operations performed under general anaesthesia, the amount of anaesthetic given is such that the patient is beginning to regain consciousness before leaving the theatre. This precaution is taken because, until the cough reflex returns, there is danger that blood may be inhaled and cause asphyxia or pneumonia. Until the patient is fully conscious, his head should be placed so that his tongue falls forward, leaving the airway clear so that vomit, mucus or blood drain freely from the mouth. To maintain a free airway by preventing the tongue from falling back into the pharynx, the nurse should place her thumb, or first and second fingers, behind the angle of the patient's jaw and pull the jaw forward.

Before leaving the table the patient is placed in the so-called 'Tonsillectomy position'. He is turned on his right side, the lower (i.e. right) knee is drawn up to form a supporting wedge and his right arm brought beneath his chin (see Fig. 13.4). This position is maintained until the patient regains consciousness.

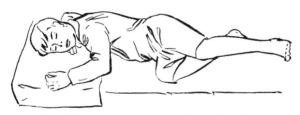

Fig. 13.4. *Post-anaesthetic (tonsillectomy) position.*

The nurse in charge of the patient must keep a constant watch until consciousness has fully returned. She should notice his colour, breathing and pulse, keeping a quarter-hourly pulse chart. Noisy breathing denotes obstruction; cyanosis indicates a deficiency of oxygen; pallor, a rapid pulse; and swallowing movements, bleeding. Should an artificial airway have been left in the mouth by the anaesthetist, this should not be removed until the patient is fully conscious.

The danger of shallow breathing should also be remembered as an important item to be observed by the nurse in charge of an anaesthetized patient. This condition, coupled with a slight degree of obstruction may lead to a state of dangerous anoxaemia (lack of oxygen in the blood). The treatment is to check the airway and give an inhalation of oxygen.

The nurse should realize that hearing is the last sense to disappear under anaesthetic and the first to return. Conversation should therefore be cautious and any remarks encouraging — for example, that the patient was very good or that the operation was successful.

14 Nursing techniques relating to the nose

Cleansing the nostrils

Once a child has learnt to blow his nose, mechanical cleansing of the nostrils is unnecessary in health. Occasionally crusts may be present inside the nose when there is local disease. These may require softening with warmed liquid paraffin, the nostrils being subsequently swabbed with warmed normal saline.

The swabs are well moistened and held in nasal forceps. Before treatments on the nose the patient should blow it.

Insertion of nasal drops

These are ordered chiefly when vasoconstriction is required, ephedrine 0.5% in normal saline being the common solution, or tuamine sulphate 0.5%. A glass dropper with a rounded end and a thin rubber bulb is convenient—if the dropper is incorporated in the stopper of the bottle containing the fluid, care should be taken that it is replaced immediately without contamination. The fluid should be slightly warmed before insertion. The patient may sit with his head forward while the drops are being inserted and should tilt his chin up, but not too far; otherwise the drops run down the floor of the nose into the pharynx and are swallowed. Usually, however, he is placed on his back, with a pillow under his shoulders, his neck straight, and his head well back (see Fig. 14.1). He should be told to breathe through the mouth. While drops are being instilled into one nostril, the other is compressed with a finger.

To supplement the use of drops, pledgets of cotton wool dipped in the lotion may be inserted under the middle conchae and left for a short time.

Spraying the nose

The apparatus used is a nasal or throat spray, the glass part of which

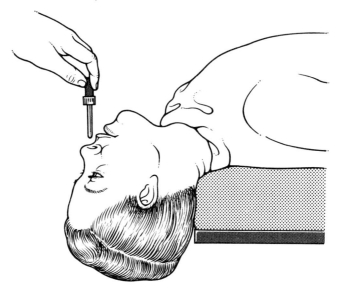

Fig. 14.1. *Position of patient for insertion of nasal drops.*

must be sterilized. After filling the spray with lotion and expelling the air, the patient's head should be held forward over a receiver and the nozzle inserted into the nostril. By gently compressing the rubber bulb, the fluid is injected with very slight force and is allowed to flow down the other nostril. It is important that the patient should breathe through the mouth whilst this is being done.

Oily fluids and antiseptic solutions are seldom used for nasal drops and sprays. Oil may be inspired into the lungs and cause pneumonia. Antiseptics, water and strong salt solutions have been found to interfere with ciliary action. The isotonic saline solution of ephedrine, previously recommended (p. 109), has no harmful effect on the ciliary movement and flow of mucus.

Packing the nose

The nose may require packing:

1. To arrest obstinate haemorrhage, when the procedure is usually performed by a doctor using gauze impregnated with bismuth and iodoform paste. A cocaine spray is applied before packing.

2. To anaesthetize it before operation or examination, when the responsibility generally rests with the surgeon performing the operation or examination. The manner in which the nose is packed may make all the difference between a comparatively painless operation and one associated with discomfort and delay. Ribbon gauze, 13 mm wide, with a selvedge, is the material used for plugging, and two pieces, each 1 m long are required. Each nostril should be packed with one piece only. If more are used, there is danger that one piece may be left behind when the packing is removed. This would set up irritation, infection and possibly ulceration.

Requirements

1. Sterile gallipot containing 8 ml of a 10% cocaine solution in which the two lengths of ribbon gauze are soaked. (Cocaine is a controlled drug. The amount must be prescribed by a doctor and checked by a competent person. Some surgeons may order a larger amount of a weaker solution, e.g. 30 ml of 5% cocaine.)
2. Gauze plugging.
3. Nasal forceps.
4. Dissecting forceps.
5. Dressed wool carriers.
6. Scissors.
7. Sterile wool swabs.
8. Receiver.

Method. The patient is seated facing a good light. The nurse puts on her mask, washes and dries her hands, and prepares the dressing trolley with the above apparatus. She washes her hands again, dries them on a clean towel, and returns to assist the doctor. The patient should be given the receiver, and told to spit out any fluid which may find its way into his throat. The doctor, using the nasal forceps, picks up the end of the plugging, which should be soaked in, but not dripping with, the cocaine solution. While supporting the other end of the plugging with dissecting forceps, he carries the first end into the nostril straight along the floor of the nose to the back of the nasal cavity. The nostril is packed firmly and gently, passing the plugging under the inferior turbinate and then under the middle turbinate bone. The other nostril is then packed in the same way. The doctor should avoid the packing being pushed into the nasopharynx and swallowed. (See Fig. 14.2.)

To obtain the full effect of the cocaine, the above procedure should be carried out 15 minutes before the operation.

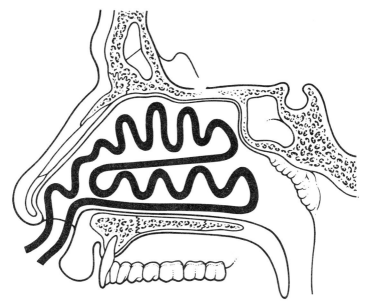

Fig. 14.2. *Anterior nasal pack.*

Another method of anaesthetizing the nose is to smear 10 or 25% cocaine paste over the mucous membrane lining the nasal cavity. The paste is commonly issued in screw-cap tubes and is applied by means of wool carriers. The carriers are inserted into each nostril and held in position for 20 minutes by a piece of adhesive strapping fixed below them, the ends reaching the bridge of the nose.

Suction displacement therapy

Conditions of chronic maxillary sinusitis present difficulties of treatment, due to the anatomical structure of the maxilla. It is possible, however, to admit fluid to the sinus, by applying suction to the nose when the patient's head is in such a position that the opening of the sinus is below the level of the fluid. The result is that air is drawn from the cavity, and the fluid replaces it.

Method. The patient lies on his back with a pillow under his shoulders, his neck straight and his head well back (as in Fig. 14.1, p. 110). A Dakin or Proetz syringe is required, and about 5 ml of warm lotion — usually 0.5% ephedrine or tuamine sulphate in normal saline. The patient is told to breathe through his mouth and to continue saying 'Kick, kick, kick'. This raises his soft palate and shuts off his nasal cavities. Whilst one nostril is being treated, the other is closed with a finger. The end of the syringe is kept inside the nose, the rubber bulb is squeezed while the patient says 'Kick' and released when he stops to breathe. This is done two or three times. The patient may then rest and sit up. He may mop excessive fluid from his upper lip, but should not blow his nose.

Steam inhalations

The periodic inhalation of steam is a treatment much used in the relief of sinusitis and other respiratory infections. There are on the market specially shaped earthenware inhalers with separate mouth-pieces of glass or earthenware (useful only for throat and chest treatment), but for most purposes in nose and throat work a 1-litre jug with a wide top is preferable. An astringent drug is usually vaporized and inhaled in the steam. Some commonly prescribed preparations are:

1. Compound tincture of benzoin (friar's balsam), 5 ml to 600 ml of water.
2. Menthol crystals, 1 or 2 ml to 600 ml of water.

In order to avoid scalding the patient's throat, and to obtain the maximum effect of the vapour, the water for the inhalation should be at a temperature of 71°C (160°F).

Requirements. A tray containing:

1. The inhalant in an airtight bottle.
2. Teaspoon, or measure.
3. Lotion thermometer.

4. Jug containing 600 ml of water at 71°C (160°F), covered with a wool or flannel bag, and standing in a bowl.

5. Towel to twist round the top of the jug to prevent the steam escaping into the room.

Method. The patient is first made to blow his nose. If he is up, he should sit at a table, on which the inhalation tray is placed. If in bed, he is best sitting with his back well supported by pillows. A patient who is unable to sit up may be treated in the lateral position. No very ill or very young patient should be left during an inhalation. The tray is brought to the patient's side, and the prescribed amount of the inhalant is floated on the water, so that none of the vapour is lost. The jug in the bowl is given to him and placed so that he can bend his head and inhale the steam without effort.

If the patient is sitting in bed a pillow may be placed over his knees. Sometimes it is considered an advantage to cover the patient's head and the jug with a bath towel. Certainly it may help the patient to concentrate on the treatment in process, but the nurse cannot then observe her patient so easily. A better method is to fold a towel in tubular form round the rim of the jug. The patient can then hold the upper edge of the towel to fit round the nose and mouth and thus avoid steaming the face and head. The patient is told to breathe in and out through the mouth for about ten minutes. In most conditions for which inhalation is prescribed, the nasal passages are closed by swollen mucous membrane, so that breathing through them is impossible. Often this treatment opens up the passages.

When the inhalation is finished, the patient's face is dried, his hair is combed, and he is covered with the bedclothes. Patients must be warned not to expose themselves to cold air for at least half an hour, and preferably for two hours after inhalation.

If a Nelson's or a Maw's inhaler is used, the water is allowed up to the lower border of the air inlet only. This precaution is taken partly to prevent spilling and partly so that the steam is driven freely from the surface of the fluid. The mouthpiece is fitted into the inhaler in such a way that the air-inlet will point away from the patient, who holds the mouthpiece, which may be covered with a layer of gauze, between his lips. After use, the mouthpiece is washed and then boiled for five minutes. The fluid used for an inhalation is poured away and the jug or inhaler is cleaned and dried. Should tincture of benzoin have been used, stains are easily removed with a swab moistened in methylated spirit.

IV The Pharynx

15   Anatomy of the pharynx

The nose and mouth open into the pharynx, which is the common passage for food and air leading to the oesophagus and the larynx. The pharynx is divided into the nasopharynx, the oropharynx and the laryngeal pharynx.

The nasopharynx

The nasopharynx lies above the soft palate and has five openings; the two posterior nares, the orifices of the two pharyngotympanic (Eustachian) tubes, and the opening downward into the oropharynx. The pharyngotympanic tubes are composed of cartilage lined by mucous membrane and at each orifice is a prominent bulge of the same tissues (see Fig. 1.1, p. 4). On the roof of the nasopharynx in childhood, and sometimes persisting into adult life, is the pharyngeal tonsil, which, if enlarged, is known as adenoids.

The oropharynx

The oropharynx lies between the soft palate and the upper edge of the epiglottis. It opens above into the nasopharynx, below into the laryngeal pharynx, and anteriorly to the mouth. The fauces separate the oropharynx from the mouth and consist of the soft palate and uvula above, and two folds on either side extending from the soft palate to the tongue, called the anterior and posterior pillars of the fauces. The faucial tonsils lie between the anterior and posterior pillars. (See Fig. 15.1.)

The laryngeal pharynx

The laryngeal pharynx runs from the level of the epiglottis to the lower border of the cricoid cartilage. Its anterior wall presents from above down towards the inlet to the larynx and the posterior surfaces of the arytenoid and cricoid cartilages. Behind this, the pharynx leads into the oesophagus.

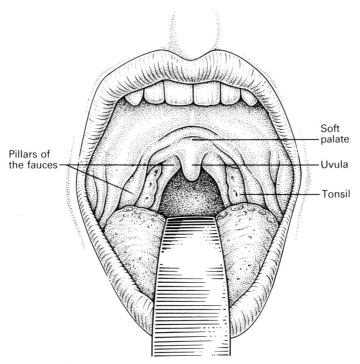

Fig. 15.1. *Looking into the mouth with the tongue depressed.*

The pharynx as a whole is a muscular tube without a front wall and is a potential space only. Its muscles originate in the side walls of the nose, mouth and larynx, and meet behind, in front of the second to the sixth cervical vertebrae. These muscles are in three groups: the superior, middle and inferior constrictors, and they contract during swallowing and push the food on. They are supplied by branches of the vagus nerve. The glossopharyngeal nerve (ninth cranial nerve) supplies the mucous membrane of the pharynx with sensory branches.

The lymphoid tissue of the pharynx

There are superficial masses of the lymphoid tissue in the pharyngeal mucosa which form a ring that acts as a filter, protecting the body against infecting organisms that might enter it from the nose or mouth. This ring of lymphoid tissue, 'Waldeyer's ring' (Fig. 15.2), consists of the *faucial or palatine tonsils*, the *pharyngeal tonsil*, the *lingual tonsil* (which lies at the back of the tongue, immediately above the epiglottis) and scattered *lymphoid nodules* occurring on the posterior and lateral walls of the pharynx. This tissue appears to aid in the production of immunity, for it increases normally during childhood, when immunity is being acquired. Except in the presence

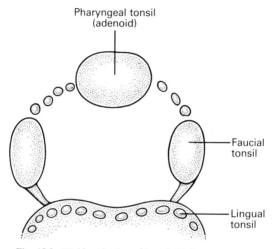

Fig. 15.2. *Waldeyer's ring of lymphoid tissue.*

of chronic infection, the pharyngeal lymphoid tissue begins to atrophy at about the time of puberty.

The pharyngeal tonsil lies on the roof and upper posterior wall of the nasopharynx. It contains many tubular crypts extending from the surface. Its surface has five or more fissures running from front to back, the lymphoid follicles being arranged along the sides of these fissures and crypts. There is no defined fibrous tissue capsule separating the pharyngeal tonsil from the superior constrictor muscle, so that complete surgical removal of all lymphoid tissue is not possible during adenoidectomy, and regrowth frequently occurs.

The faucial tonsils consist of lymphoid tissue with 8–20 tubular crypts, which frequently branch in the depth of the tonsil (Fig. 15.3). Whereas the adenoid is covered with ciliated mucous membrane

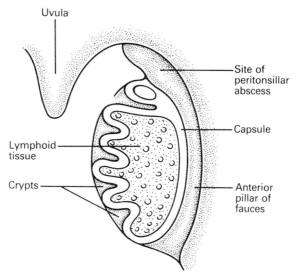

Fig. 15.3. *The faucial tonsil.*

which keeps the fissures swept clean of debris, the faucial tonsil is covered with stratified squamous epithelium, and desquamated epithelial cells and lymphocytes normally collect in the crypts. The faucial tonsil is enclosed in a capsule which enables complete enucleation of all tonsillar material by splitting the capsule.

The lymphatics of the pharynx are numerous, and drain into the anterior cervical glands, in front of the sternomastoid muscle, except those from the nasopharynx and posterior oropharynx, some of which drain into the posterior cervical lymph glands, behind the same muscle.

16 Diseases of the throat

ACUTE INFLAMMATIONS

Acute inflammation of the throat is a distressingly common condition, of which the chief symptom is soreness. The tonsils are particularly likely to be involved in the infection and the tonsillitis then overshadows the adjacent inflammation.

Causes. The causes of inflammation are:

1. Haemolytic streptococci, though other organisms usually found in the throat, such as *Streptococcus viridans*, pneumococci, *Neisseria catarrhalis*, and viruses, may be increased in such infection.
2. Staphylococci, especially in the summer.
3. *Corynebacterium diphtheriae.*
4. Vincent's infection — an association of a spirillum and a fusiform bacillus.
5. Thrush, caused by *Candida albicans.*
6. Syphilis.
7. Blood diseases, such as acute leukaemia and agranulocytic angina.

Streptococcal sore throat (acute follicular tonsillitis)

Signs and Symptoms. This infection is abrupt in onset and usually occurs when the victim's resistance is lowered by fatigue, chilling or coryza. The inflammation is concentrated in the faucial tonsils and penetrates deeply into the mucous membrane. On inspection, the uvula is seen to be inflamed and thickened, the tonsils are red and swollen and there are spots of yellowish exudate from the tonsillar crypts. The anterior cervical glands, below the angle of the jaw, are enlarged and tender. There may be continuous pain at the back of the throat, with a sensation of rawness, or the patient may complain of severe pain only on swallowing. The temperature rises sharply to 39°C (102°F), or higher, and the initial rise may be accompanied by rigor.

In the course of a severe infection, ulceration of the tonsil surface occurs, and patches of exudate form a membrane which is distinguishable from diphtheria in that it can be detached. Diagnosis is confirmed by culture from a throat swab.

Complications. Occasionally ulceration in the depths of the crypts leads to the formation of thrombi in the vessels at the base of the tonsils. This results in systemic infections such as acute nephritis, arthritis and rheumatic fever, with or without cardiac involvement. Symptoms of these complications appear after the sore throat and pyrexia have abated. If nephritis develops, albuminuria is found in the third week from the onset of the tonsillitis. Other complications that are liable to follow acute follicular tonsillitis, especially in the young, are extensions of the inflammation upward, or to the ears, or downward to the larynx. Oedema may be so great as to obstruct respiration and swallowing.

Treatment. Acute streptococcal tonsillitis is generally a self-limiting disease and will subside in a few days.

The patient should be confined to bed and isolated to prevent droplet infection. Hot gargles of sodium bicarbonate, or other mild lotions, may be used. However, since the effort of gargling sometimes increases the pain, and the lotion does not reach the whole of the inflamed area, the treatment is not always useful. Treatment by throat spray with an appropriate antibiotic is generally preferred. The sucking of lozenges keeps up the salivary secretion and tends to prevent stiffness of the neck muscles. Many varieties of lozenge dispensed for this purpose contain such drugs as phenol and ammonium bromide.

Four-hourly steam inhalations with menthol or tincture of benzoin compound are commonly ordered.

The diet is necessarily fluid at the onset of tonsillitis, when the temperature is high, swallowing difficult and the throat raw. It may be difficult to persuade the patient to drink enough, but he must be encouraged to take from four to five litres daily. Lemon drink, orangeade and barley water are generally much appreciated and should be alternated with milk variously flavoured. Fluids can be made highly nourishing by the addition of glucose, lactose, Ovaltine, malted milk, chocolate, or beaten egg, according to the patient's taste. The doctor may order additional vitamins. As soon as the patient is capable of taking more substantial food, his appetite should be tempted. A child may be helped in swallowing if the nurse supports his neck with her hands as he makes the effort. Ice cream is often acceptable and soft solids may be swallowed more easily than liquids.

Frequent mouth-washes are necessary, and should be given before and after any food or milk drink. Since the patient is confined to bed whilst fever is present, pressure areas require regular treatment and a daily bed-bath should be given at this stage. The bedclothes should be light and applied according to the patient's comfort.

A four-hourly temperature record should be kept, the urine tested daily, and the fluid intake and output measured.

Chemotherapy is the rule, and with it, the inflammation usually dies down after four or five days. The patient is toxaemic, if not septicaemic, and after an acute attack of tonsillitis, suffers from weakness and fatigue for a few weeks. The chief principles to observe in order to lessen this debility are rest and nourishment. The patient is advised to avoid strenuous exercise for several days after the temperature has returned to normal. After haemolytic streptococcal infection, an iron preparation may be prescribed by the doctor.

The nurse should observe the patient for any signs of systemic complications. The first signs of acute nephritis are early morning oedema of the face, backs of the hands or ankles, and a diminished urinary output with albuminuria.

Any return of fever or complaint of pain in the joints should be reported to the doctor.

Acute pharyngitis

Acute pharyngitis caused by haemolytic streptococci in patients who have had their tonsils removed is seldom as severe an inflammation as that of acute follicular tonsillitis, but follows a similar course and may have the same complications. The inflammation begins in the nasopharynx and travels to the laryngeal pharynx or vice versa. The mucous membrane shows varying degrees of redness, and in the areas where tonsils have been removed, bright patches of lymphoid tissue are often seen. Exudate from these may become membranous as in tonsillitis, and other signs and symptoms are similar.

Treatment follows the same lines as for tonsillitis, although the patient is not usually acutely ill and the temperature is only mildly raised.

Recurrent attacks of acute pharyngitis need investigation. This may be caused by an allergic condition, or an infective focus such as adenoids, infected tonsils or tonsils incompletely removed.

Scarlet fever (scarlatina)

This is an acute pharyngitis or tonsillitis accompanied by a skin rash. The cause is a haemolytic streptococcus of a special type which produces a toxin capable of causing the rash, though no rash occurs if the patient is already immune to the specific toxin. Confusion can occur between the diagnosis of acute tonsillitis and scarlet fever. Both types are equally infectious, and a victim of acute follicular tonsillitis may be much more ill than one with an extensive scarlet rash. However, scarlet fever is a notifiable disease, and the patient is nursed in isolation.

As scarlet fever is more common in childhood, before immunity is great, local complications such as otitis media, sinusitis and suppurative adenitis of the neck may occur, as well as systemic infection. Fortunately the incidence of scarlet fever is decreasing.

Peritonsillar abscess ('quinsy')

This is an abscess in the cellular tissue outside the tonsil capsule, between it and the constrictor muscles of the pharynx. After repeated attacks of tonsillitis, an intratonsillar abscess in the depths of a stenosed crypt bursts laterally through the tonsil capsule.

Signs and symptoms. After a few days of tonsillitis, the patient experiences increasing pain on one side and increasing difficulty in swallowing. He holds his head stiffly towards the side of the abscess and is obviously in distressing pain. His throat is red and there is marked swelling of the soft palate on the side of the abscess, with displacement of the uvula to the opposite side. The tonsil itself is displaced toward the midline (see Fig. 16.1). The glands below the angle of the jaw are enlarged and tender, but there is usually not much fever.

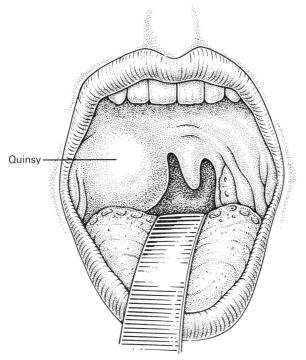

Quinsy

Fig. 16.1. *'Quinsy' or peritonsillar abscess.*

Complications of which the nurse should be aware are a downward spread of the infection, oedema of the glottis and thrombophlebitis of one of the large veins in the neck.

Treatment. In addition to the treatment of the preceding tonsillitis, the patient should be provided with a sputum container, since he may be unable to swallow his saliva.

When a rounded bulge indicates that the accumulated pus has become localized, the abscess is incised and drained, generally under a local anaesthetic. Antibiotic therapy is usually continued until the inflammation has subsided completely, or until the course is completed, whichever takes longer. At this stage, whilst the patient's immunity is still high and before scar tissue has become dense, tonsillectomy is generally performed. Otherwise a recurrence of the quinsy is highly probable.

Retropharyngeal abscess

This is a collection of pus between the posterior pharyngeal wall and the vertebrae. There are two types of abscess, acute and chronic.

1. The acute form

The acute form is due to an infection in lymph glands situated on each side of the pharynx, superficial to the prevertebral fascia. These glands atrophy early in childhood, and therefore a retropharyngeal abscess of this type occurs only in infancy. The suppuration is usually one-sided.

Symptoms. The illness may follow an upper respiratory infection such as coryza or measles. The degree of fever is variable. The chief symptom is difficulty of swallowing. The child refuses to feed or the food is regurgitated. As the abscess spreads downwards, dyspnoea and inspiratory stridor develop, owing to the narrowing of the airway. The child is extremely ill—restless, sweating, cyanosed and sometimes vomiting—and unless prompt treatment is instituted, the case ends fatally. An X-ray of the neck helps the diagnosis.

Complications. The chief dangers are respiratory obstruction and haemorrhage from the internal carotid artery. If dyspnoea is present, the mouth must not be forcibly opened with a gag, lest this should cause the abscess to rupture suddenly and the septic material to be inhaled.

Treatment. When diagnosis of retropharyngeal abscess is made, suction apparatus should be immediately procured. The abscess is incised, using as a rule a guarded scalpel. This procedure is usually carried out without anaesthetic, with the child firmly wrapped in a blanket, lying on his back, with his head low. Then, as pus appears, he is turned quickly on to his abdomen, with his head and shoulders over the edge of the table. Suction should be used as required. Tracheotomy instruments are kept at hand during and after the operation. Recovery is generally rapid. The incision should be kept open daily by the insertion of artery forceps until no more pus escapes.

Haemorrhage from the carotid artery requires prompt ligation of the artery to avoid a recurrence. A child usually recovers from a first haemorrhage, but seldom survives a second. At the first warning — a few spots of blood coughed up — the nurse should immediately inform the surgeon.

2. *The chronic form*

The chronic form of retropharyngeal abscess is due to tuberculosis of the bodies of the cervical vertebrae and occurs in older children and adults. The abscess causes bulging, often bilateral, of the posterior pharyngeal wall.

Both types of abscess are extremely dangerous. The head is held stiffly and there are violent pains, especially at night. The abscess is opened through an external incision behind the sternomastoid muscle.

Faucial diphtheria

Where immunization in infancy and childhood is universal, the disease has been almost completely wiped out. Such cases as occur in immunized persons are comparatively mild, and the early administration of antitoxin prevents the serious complications.

Course and signs of the disease

An infection of the throat by the *Corynebacterium diphtheriae* is likely to be a much more serious condition than the nasal diphtheria described in Chapter 11. It is transmitted in the same way — that is, by direct contact or from carriers harbouring the bacilli in the pharynx. The organisms settle in the tonsil and produce a toxin which destroys the surface epithelium. This causes an exudate of serum which coagulates and forms a dirty grey membrane — like the surface of a cut raw potato which has been left dry. The membrane is adherent and has well-defined margins. It spreads from the tonsils to the soft palate and sometimes on to the posterior pharyngeal wall. There is a 'mousy' odour to the breath. The cervical lymph glands are enlarged and tender.

The incubation period is from two to five days. There is a gradual onset of sore throat, low-grade fever ($37.5°–38°C$, $99°–101°F$) with an increase of pulse rate out of proportion to the rise in temperature. The pulse rate is frequently 120 to 140 beats per minute. Toxaemia is marked and the patient is very ill indeed, although neither pyrexia nor sore throat are extreme. The tonsils are at first swollen and red; then the membrane appears. Speech is painful and has a nasal 'twang', the patient talking as though he held a plum in his mouth. Diagnosis is confirmed by culture from a throat swab which has been rubbed over the membrane and then on to Loeffler's medium. It is examined after 12–18 hours.

Complications. The complications that are likely to arise are due either to the spread of the inflammation into the larynx, or to the spread of the toxins. While the bacilli remain in the local area they have invaded, the toxins produced spread through the lymphatic and blood circulation to the tissues. These toxins specifically affect the heart muscle and the nervous system, causing myocardial damage and paralyses of various muscles, as for example, the soft palate, the eye muscles, the pharyngeal muscles and the diaphragm. Heart failure is the most usual cause of death from diphtheria, due to degeneration of the cardiac muscle. The most common of the paralyses is that of the soft palate, which develops in the second or third week of the disease, after the acute symptoms have subsided, and lasts two or three weeks. It causes regurgitation of fluid through the nose. Paralysis of the eye muscles will cause squinting — this too disappears in a few weeks.

Oedema of the throat and membranous obstruction may require tracheostomy.

Fortunately, the complications of diphtheria are seldom seen nowadays.

Treatment. If diphtheria is suspected, 20 000–40 000 units of anti-toxin are given immediately, without waiting for the report on the throat swab. The patient should be put to bed and isolated — usually in an isolation unit. The nursing treatment is carried out under strict isolation precautions. The nurse should be immune to diphtheria and should wear a mask and gown. The patient is nursed in the recumbent position, pillows being allowed only by the doctor's orders. He is kept at complete rest, being fed and washed by the nurse until all danger of heart complications is past. Food is at first restricted to milky fluids, and semi-solids, since condiments and acid drinks such as lemonade are painful to swallow whilst the throat is raw. Thickened milk foods, such as cornflour, egg nog and custard are easily swallowed. Reaction to the large doses of antitoxin, or 'serum sickness', should be watched for. This may give rise to fever, an urticarial rash or joint pains, and is treated symptomatically. It usually occurs one or two days after the injection. Rarely, anaphylactic shock occurs with the injection of antitoxin.

Glandular fever — infectious mononucleosis

This is an infectious disease, the causative organism of which is a virus; the incubation period is seven days. Its characteristic features are fever, enlargement of the lymphatic glands, including the tonsils, and changes in the blood. The white blood count is raised, the lymphocytes being especially increased, larger than normal and bluish. The Paul–Bunnel agglutination test is positive.

Signs and symptoms. The symptoms are malaise, headache and an unusually persistent sore throat. The cervical glands are especially affected, particularly those deep to the sternomastoid muscle, and may swell rapidly. Axillary glands are generally enlarged also. The tonsils, although red and swollen, do not produce an exudate except in those subject to tonsillitis.

Treatment. The treatment is symptomatic. Recurrences occasionally extend over several weeks, and debility may persist for many months, but recovery is the rule.

Vincent's angina

This is a specific infection of the mouth or pharynx due to the associated existence of a spirillum and a fusiform bacillus. The disease may occur in epidemics, being transmitted by direct contact, or it frequently arises from organisms already existing in the mouth, when there is lack of oral hygiene or of vitamin C.

Signs and symptoms. The first sign is a dirty-grey, punched-out ulcer usually on one tonsil. The ulceration spreads over the gums, there is soreness of throat and mouth, slight pyrexia and enlargement of the cervical glands. Sloughs form at the bottom of the ulcers, covering granulations that bleed easily. The odour of the breath is particularly offensive. The diagnosis is supported by finding fusiform bacilli and spirilla in large numbers in a smear from an ulcer.

Treatment. The patient is not usually kept in bed, nor is he isolated except for keeping separate his feeding utensils. As full a diet is given as can be taken with comfort, and large amounts of vitamin C — for example: 200 milligrams of ascorbic acid twice daily. Intramuscular injection of an antibiotic usually brings about recovery in 36 hours. The local treatment consists of mouth-washes before and after every meal or drink, together with thorough cleansing of the teeth. If a tooth-brush is used, it should be a soft one and, when not in use, should be kept in an antiseptic solution, such as sodium hypochlorite.

The patient should be examined by the doctor four days after the pyrexia and adenitis have subsided. Frequently, dental treatment is deemed necessary.

Another method of treating Vincent's angina is to paint the affected area with 5% neoarsphenamine in glycerin and then to insufflate with bismuth subnitrate powder four times a day. Since the condition is very common and is often difficult to cure, the nurse may meet a variety of treatments with different patients and different surgeons.

Fungal stomatitis ('thrush')

Thrush is stomatitis (inflammation of the mouth) or pharyngitis characterized by adherent small white patches on the mucous membrane. It is due to a fungus, commonly *Candida albicans.* Very little inflammation occurs under the patches and there are often no other symptoms — no sore throat or fever — except loss of taste and appetite. It occurs in infants on the cheeks and lips, and in adults (generally those on a milk diet) on the faucial and lingual tonsils and on the pharyngeal lymph nodes. The condition is usually considered due to neglect of oral hygiene and in the sterilization of infant feeding bottles and teats. It seldom arises in breast-fed babies.

Treatment. The treatment for an adult consists of gentle cleansing of the mouth. In addition, the doctor may prescribe nystatin suspension, or the use of lozenges. For a baby, the self-cleansing by a teaspoonful of boiled water after feeds is the only local treatment. The feeding bottles should be kept scrupulously clean. After washing, they should be boiled or immersed in a solution of sodium hypochlorite.

Syphilis of the throat

Primary syphilis — chancre of the tonsil — is extremely rare. One or two cases have been reported and have been ascribed to the use of a contaminated drinking vessel. An indurated swelling occurs, with ulceration and a sore throat which persists longer than a week. Diagnosis is made by finding the organism, the *Treponema pallidum*, in a swab taken from the ulcer.

Secondary syphilis frequently causes a sore throat, some 6–12 weeks after primary infection. The mucous membrane shows dull red areas, slightly elevated, on which are round, oval or long patches of ulceration, with defined borders and a shining, pearly surface ('snail-track' ulcers). These usually occur on the tonsils or pillars of the fauces or on the inner surface of the lips. They are accompanied by moderate, remittent pyrexia, generalized enlargement and hardness of lymph glands, and skin rashes. The organisms can be demonstrated in the blood stream, the Wassermann reaction is strongly positive and the patient at this stage is highly infectious.

Treatment. Specific antisyphilitic treatment is necessary, i.e., intramuscular injection of penicillin.

The nursing treatment consists largely of preventing the spread of infection. This can occur only by inoculation, but any abrasion of the skin or mucous membrane might allow the organisms to enter. Disposable feeding and washing utensils should be used, and the nurse should wear non-sterile disposable gloves when attending to the patient.

Agranulocytic angina

Cause. This sore throat is due to damage of the bone marrow by infection or drugs, especially by amidopyrine, gold, thyroid-suppressing drugs, some steroids, some antibiotics (particularly chloramphenicol) and sulphonamides. The agranulocytosis is more frequent when large doses of the drug are given over a long period, or when the patient has been sensitized by previous administration.

Symptoms.
1. The patient suffers from severe exhaustion.
2. Rapidly spreading ulceration occurs on the tonsils, pharynx and mouth, with pain.

3. A white blood cell count, which is diagnostic, shows a diminution or absence of polymorphonuclear leucocytes. The total white cell count is low — for example, 2000 per cubic millimetre of blood.
4. Fever is slight in mild cases, severe in acute ones.
5. Jaundice may occur, or cyanosis in sulphonamide poisoning.
6. Haemorrhage sometimes arises from the ulcers.
7. Death may occur within a few days from the onset of the ulceration.

Treatment. The drug responsible for the condition must be discontinued. Large doses of an antibiotic, and a transfusion of packed cells or blood, may be given. In successful cases, the leucocyte count begins to return to normal about five days after the treatment commences.

Local treatment of the sore throat is required — in particular, frequent mouth-washes and anaesthetic lozenges.

Acute leukaemia

In acute leukaemia there is a permanent increase in the number of white blood cells. These excess cells are abnormal and have no protective function. The cause is the subject of much research.

The tonsils may be red, swollen and ulcerated. The glands are generally enlarged. There is sore throat, fever, haemorrhage from the mucous membranes, and a rapidly progressive anaemia.

The treatment is symptomatic as there is no known cure at present.

CHRONIC DISEASES OF THE PHARYNX

Chronic tonsillitis

This usually follows an acute attack of tonsillitis caused by haemolytic streptococci.

Signs. The tonsils and the anterior pillars of the fauces are persistently reddened. The tonsils may be enlarged or may be small and fibrous, and collect an abnormal amount of caseous debris in their crypts. Ulceration occurs in the depths of the crypts and liquid pus can generally be expressed from them on slight pressure from a spatula. Sometimes the crypts are sealed off, and then small abscesses result.

Local symptoms. These include mild soreness, with recurrent attacks of acute inflammation, an unpleasant-tasting exudate from the tonsils and discomfort located in the cervical glands.

General symptoms. Loss of appetite, chronic fatigue, acute and chronic arthritis, fibrositis, neuritis, iritis and other subacute infections occur, for which the diseased tonsils act as a focus.
   The only satisfactory treatment is tonsillectomy.

Adenoids

The pharyngeal tonsil normally reaches its maximum development in mid-childhood, then atrophies and disappears at puberty. With chronic infection, enlargements of the tissue, termed 'adenoids', may occur, and they frequently persist into adult life.

Local symptoms. These are mouth-breathing, snoring and frequent, prolonged head colds, due to nasal obstruction. They lead to sinusitis with a typical copious nasal discharge, or to recurrent or chronic suppurative otitis media when the pharyngotympanic (Eustachian) tubes are infected. Defective hearing may become permanent deafness due to blockage of the tubes.

General symptoms. These are the same as for chronic tonsillitis.

Treatment. This is at first conservative, by correction of diet, plenty of fresh air and exercise and by breathing exercises. Should the adenoid tissue enlarge to reach the upper level of the posterior nares, adenoidectomy is performed. In most cases, all symptoms then disappear spontaneously, and children improve both in appearance and in mental capacity.
   Hyperplasia of lymphoid tissue in children may be treated with small doses of deep X-rays when the condition has not been relieved by adenoidectomy or has recurred.

Chronic pharyngitis

A chronic inflammation of the pharynx, without the formation of ulcers, may result from allergy, alcohol or smoking, or be an extension of atrophic rhinitis or sinusitis, or accompany metabolic diseases such as anaemia, diabetes or gout.

Signs. The signs are a diffuse redness, the enlargement of superficial lymph nodules, dryness of the throat and sometimes crusting, especially of the nasopharynx. There is a sense of irritation, soreness at times, with slight discomfort on swallowing.

Treatment. The treatment is directed towards the general health, and the cause is removed if known. Smoking should be avoided.

Tuberculous pharyngitis

This condition is secondary to pulmonary tuberculosis. Irregular, shallow ulcers with pale granulations can be seen in the pharynx and there is pain on swallowing. Signs of general tuberculosis, such as fatigue, wasting and evening pyrexia are present. Treatment of the lung condition must be instituted, and with its improvement, the pharyngitis clears up.

Syphilitic pharyngitis

With tertiary syphilis, gumma may appear in the pharynx, causing, as elsewhere, painless swellings, with a tendency to ulcerate and to heal with much scarring. Perforations of the palate or of the faucial pillars may result.

General treatment of syphilis is required, local applications having little effect.

Actinomycosis

This disease is caused by the 'ray fungus', a vegetable parasite which occasionally attacks the pharynx. It causes a firm, painless swelling, which proceeds to ulceration and suppuration, the discharge containing the distinctive yellow 'sulphur granules'.

Treatment. The treatment is to give iodides internally, Lugol's iodine being frequently prescribed. (N.B. Lugol's iodine should always be given in milk, to avoid staining of the teeth.) A prolonged course of an antibiotic has also proved effective.

NEW GROWTHS OF THE PHARYNX

Benign new growths

A *papilloma* most often grows from the base of the uvula and is pedunculated.

An *adenoma* is rare. It occurs in the uvula or soft palate, and forms a firm swelling under the mucous membrane.

A *fibroma* occurs as a rounded growth, most often on the posterior pharyngeal wall.

All the above tumours can be removed surgically.

Haemangiomata are sometimes found on the posterior pharyngeal wall. They are bluish, and may be sessile or pedunculated. They bleed easily when touched. The treatment is by cauterization or by radiotherapy.

Malignant new growths

These rarely occur before forty years of age.

Carcinoma may involve any part, but chiefly the lower lateral pharyngeal wall.

Carcinoma and sarcoma of the tonsil

Both types of new growth of the tonsil occur. If a unilateral enlargement, which is inflamed, does not respond to local treatment, biopsy should be done. A malignant growth develops rapidly into an ulcer with a hard irregular edge. In early cases there is no enlargement of glands, but glands at the angle of the jaw are occasionally the first sign of the disease.

Symptoms. The symptoms are proportional to the extent of the lesion. If the pillars, the tongue and the posterior pharyngeal wall are involved, there is difficulty in swallowing. The movements of the tongue are restricted. The patient complains of pain radiating to the ear. Later, excessive mucus occurs, occasionally some bleeding, and more pain. When the new growth is confined to the tonsil, the prognosis is good.

Treatment. Radiotherapy is particularly successful in this type of malignancy, but radical dissection of secondarily invaded glands may be needed.

Carcinoma of the lower pharynx

This usually occurs behind the cricoid cartilage in women or in the piriform fossa in men. It is a firm, elevated growth, which breaks down in the centre, leaving an ulcerated area with a crater-like indurated rim.

Symptoms. The symptoms vary from a vague discomfort, such as a sensation of fulness, to pain extending to the ear. There is rapid invasion of the adjacent tissue and glands, so that an early diagnosis is imperative for cure.

Treatment. Piriform fossa lesions do reasonably well on radiotherapy, but the glands usually need surgery. Post-cricoid cases are rarely affected by radiotherapy and radical surgery provides the only hope.

Growths of the nasopharynx are rare but occasionally the pharyngotympanic tube may be blocked by a growth. Radiotherapy or the insertion of radium is usually indicated. An operation has been devised in which a transpalatal incision is made where the soft palate joins the hard palate. The soft palate then drops down and the nasopharynx can be explored, in order to establish a diagnosis or to remove a benign tumour.

17 Tonsillectomy and adenoidectomy

In childhood, these two operations for removal of the tonsils and adenoids are commonly performed together as treatment for chronic inflammation. In adult life, tonsillectomy is frequently all that is needed, the adenoids having atrophied. The operation usually takes place a few weeks after the occurrence of sore throat. It is contraindicated in the presence of an acute infection (especially of the respiratory tract) or blood disease such as haemophilia or anaemia. The patient is admitted to hospital at least one day before operation.

The two chief methods of removing tonsils are:

Enucleation by guillotine. This operation is a rapid one and very satisfactory in skilled hands. It is particularly popular when there are large numbers of patients to be treated, but is normally only used with children or the small adult.

Enucleation by dissection. This is essential for long-standing inflammation and after peritonsillar abscess.

Preparation of a child for hospital treatment

The psychological effect on a small child of a period in hospital depends a great deal upon the age and emotional development of the child and upon the preparation given by his parents before admission. The duration in hospital for tonsillectomy is short and the subjects are usually of the age to accept a brief explanation of what is to be expected. Being a patient in hospital can be a valuable and is often an enjoyable experience, but children need preparation to face what is strange and unpleasant. Parents can be given guidance on how to help their children and frequently need reassurance themselves. Many hospitals issue leaflets of information and advice to parents of children awaiting admission and sometimes a separate welcoming leaflet is given to the child himself. Recent research has shown that most school children whose views were asked had fear of operations and anaesthetics. Some of those who had been patients emphasized the fears they had had before operation rather than any postoperative experiences.

When possible, the mother should bring her child to the ward, help him undress, and stay for as long as she is able. Some hospitals have mother and child units, and, when family circumstances allow, the mother may remain in hospital with the child. A young child should be allowed to keep a favourite toy or possession. There should be mutual understanding between parents and nursing staff and arrangements should be made for telephone enquiries, visiting and fetching the child home.

Preoperative treatment

The procedure following the admission of the patient follows the usual routine. The history of the patient is taken and the throat, heart and lungs are examined. The urine is tested and, if necessary, the bleeding and clotting times are estimated. Apart from attention to the cleanliness of the mouth and the removal of dentures if worn, no preparation of the throat is required. The meal before operation is omitted. Children are usually given a sedative such as pentobarbitone sodium (Nembutal) or trimeprazine tartrate (Vallergan syrup) an hour or more before operation, and oral atropine, the dose varying according to the child's weight. Otherwise, premedication before general anaesthesia is prescribed by the anaesthetist.

The guillotine operation

As soon as the child is under the anaesthetic the mouth is opened widely with a gag such as Doyen's. A guillotine, for example Heath's or Ballenger's, is used, and the tonsil is pushed by the surgeon's finger through the ring of the guillotine, the blade is pushed home and the tonsil is peeled off by the surgeon's forefinger. If necessary, the adenoids are then removed with a curette and the patient is turned on his face so that the blood runs out of his mouth. Bleeding quickly ceases. The surgeon inspects the throat, the anaesthetist satisfies himself that the cough reflex has returned, and the child is placed on a trolley and returned to the ward.

Dissection of tonsils

There are many methods of performing this operation and almost every throat specialist has his preferences regarding his own position, the patient's position, the instruments used and the technique followed. The main differences in procedure are: blunt dissection, using long-bladed dissecting forceps, and sharp dissection, using scissors. Some surgeons combine the two. The aim is to dissect the tonsil in the plane of its capsule and ensure that it is completely removed. The dissection is carried below the lower pole of the palatine tonsil, to exclude the lingual tonsil, which extends along the base of the tongue. If diseased tonsil remnants are left, they are apt to cause further trouble. Even after a thorough tonsillectomy, lymphoid tissue occasionally enlarges and tonsillitis recurs.

Operation under general anaesthesia

The choice of anaesthetic depends upon the agreement of surgeon and anaesthetist. As soon as relaxation occurs, the patient's head is placed in the desired position for operation. If suction is used during operation, no aspiration of blood will occur. A mouth gag is inserted, of a type such as Davis's, with a small, medium or large tongue blade according to the size of the patient. The gag is opened and rubber tubing which connects with the vaporizer is attached to the metal tube. The surgeon takes up his position and his head lamp is adjusted. The suction tube is placed ready at hand, and the instrument table on his left.

Some surgeons remove adenoids (if present) first, so that the bleeding from the nasopharynx will have ceased before the patient returns to bed. With his gloved finger, the operator feels for the enlarged tissue behind the palate. Then, using a La Force adenotome or a guarded curette, the adenoids are gently swept off in one piece. A small gauze pack 25 mm by 38 mm, tied with a length of tape is inserted into the nasopharynx, with the tape hanging out of the mouth, and left until the completion of the operation.

For tonsillectomy, the tonsil is drawn forward by a volsellum or special tonsil-holding forceps, and then it is dissected from its bed. Frequent mopping or suction is required to keep the pharynx clear of blood. Bleeding points are picked up and ligated with linen thread. Suturing is rarely needed, but if so, the stitch should be removed the following day. Sometimes, each tonsil fossa is packed for a short time with a mop soaked in adrenaline solution. The post-nasal pack is removed and a final inspection is made to see that no gauze mops are left behind, and a count is made. The patient is then turned well over on his side. The coughing and swallowing reflexes must have returned before the patient may leave the theatre. The anaesthetist will give clear oral and written instructions to the ward nurse regarding the patient's immediate postoperative care. Any postoperative analgesia will be prescribed by the anaesthetist before the patient leaves the theatre area.

Postoperative treatment of tonsillectomy

The outstanding aim is to maintain a clear airway and prevent asphyxia from inhaled blood and blood clots. Sips of water are allowed as soon as the patient is awake, and when vomiting has ceased, he is encouraged to swallow. This prevents stiffness of the pharyngeal muscles, and militates against infection. The more the patient swallows, the easier it becomes. An aspirin mixture may be gargled and swallowed every few hours (for example, 20 minutes before meals). Children suffer comparatively little pain, and ice cream and jelly usually tempt them to swallow. A child is usually sent home on the second day if his temperature is below 37.5°C (99°F), and there is no bleeding. Adults do not recover as rapidly and it is important that they should not become dehydrated by refusing to swallow. The morning after operation, a light diet is given, and thereafter the patient is encouraged to return to an ordinary diet. A simple gargle of glycerin of thymol is given after meals. The patient is allowed out of bed on the day after operation and goes home, in normal cases, within the week.

Complications after tonsillectomy and adenoidectomy

Haemorrhage

This may be reactionary, occurring within 12 hours of operation, or secondary, occurring 5–7 days afterwards. The latter is due to sepsis. An adult is normally aware of blood on swallowing, and will indicate his concern to the nurse. A child, however, may be too young to know what is happening to him, and the nurse must watch him for excessive swallowing.

The child or adult should be sat up in bed, head and neck well supported by pillows. The nurse will then examine the tonsil beds for signs of bleeding. The patient's blood pressure and pulse should then be taken and recorded, and the surgeon informed of the patient's medical condition.

Treatment of bleeding from tonsillar fossae. The surgeon removes the clot carefully by means of Luc's forceps. He then mops the fossa with wool soaked in hydrogen peroxide. If this does not cause the bleeding to stop, it may be necessary to take the patient back to the theatre and ligate one or more vessels.

Treatment of bleeding from adenoids. It is rarely necessary to assist nature in controlling bleeding after adenoidectomy, and sitting the child up may be all that is required, but if troublesome bleeding should occur it may be treated by inserting post-nasal packs. The surgeon may first retract the uvula in order to remove a tag of adenoid tissue.

For the packs, two strips of ribbon gauze folded and tied to a size of approximately 25 mm by 38 mm by tape or linen thread, or two marine sponges, are required. A soft rubber catheter is passed along the floor of one nostril until it appears in the pharynx. It is then pulled out through the mouth sufficiently far to enable the operator to tie one of the packs to the eye end of the catheter (see Fig. 17.1). A second thread is attached to the pack and brought out through the mouth for the removal of the pack in due course. The end of the catheter protruding from the nostril is then pulled back through the nose, bringing the thread with it until further withdrawal of the thread is prevented by the lodgement of the pack in the post-nasal space. The catheter is then detached. The threads are secured to the cheeks by small pieces of adhesive tape (see Fig. 17.2).

The packing is usually left for 24 hours and then removed by cutting the thread from the nose and withdrawing the pack by the thread through the mouth. Should bleeding recur, fresh packing will be inserted. Since sepsis is likely to be present, an antibiotic is usually given to prevent infection going up the pharyngotympanic (Eustachian) tubes.

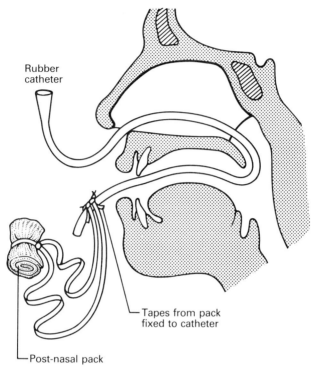

Rubber
catheter

Tapes from pack
fixed to catheter

Post-nasal pack

Fig. 17.1. *Post-nasal pack ready for introduction.*

Atelectasis (partial collapse of lung)

This complication may arise if a plug of mucus blocks one of the bronchial tubes. The signs are elevation of temperature, rapid breathing, dyspnoea, cough and cyanosis. There will be dullness in the affected side, with absence of breath sounds over the area involved. Radiographs will show that the heart is displaced toward, and the diaphragm is raised on, the collapsed side.

The patient is prepared for theatre, where a bronchoscopy is performed in order to aspirate the occluding plug.

Pneumonia

At first the clinical picture of pneumonia is the same as that of

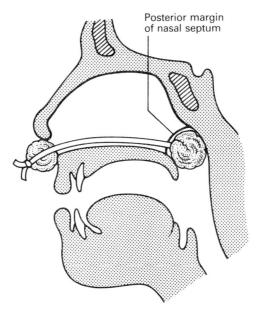

Fig. 17.2. *Post-nasal pack in position, with tapes tied across small gauze swab anteriorly. Thread through mouth not shown.*

atelectasis (above). Breath sounds, however, are increased and X-rays will show a different picture.

Lung abscess

This complication is very rare if the head is hyperextended during operation, thus preventing inhalation of any material such as blood and mucus.

The signs are elevation of temperature, cough and purulent sputum occurring one to two weeks after operation.

Discharge of a child after tonsillectomy

The child's mother is advised that strenuous exercise or play must be avoided for one week following discharge from hospital. Normal diet should be taken, some centres advising the use of chewing-gum to encourage saliva production. Crowded places, such as the cinema, should be avoided, in case the child is in contact with viral infections, etc. Should the child haemorrhage, then immediate return to hospital is essential. Special breathing exercises are sometimes recommended. These are usually taught in a physiotherapy clinic, for which the mother and child are given an appointment.

Breathing exercises after tonsillectomy and adenoidectomy

The habit of nasal speech which a child develops from enlargement of the adenoids is difficult to eliminate without perseverance. Certain exercises have been devised before which the child should blow his nose, one nostril at a time. It is essential that the mouth should be kept shut during the exercises, of which the following are examples.

1. Breathe in deeply via the nose. Breathe out slowly.
2. The arms are raised above the head whilst breathing in, and lowered on expiration. The shoulders must not be raised and the arms should be well back to expand the chest.
3. Whilst the nurse or mother keeps a hand on the child's back, the child himself should take a deep breath through the nose and try to push the hand away, at the same time pulling in his abdomen. Then he should breathe out through the nose, relaxing the abdomen.
4. Humming through the nose is amusing and beneficial. The child may think of going up a steep hill whilst breathing in and pushing hard downhill when breathing out.

These exercises should be performed two or three times daily and initially are best done in groups.

V The Larynx, Trachea and Oesophagus

18 Anatomy of the larynx, voice production and swallowing

All animal life originally was aquatic and derived oxygen from water. Lungs were therefore unnecessary. As the water receded it was necessary for animals to take oxygen from the air instead of from water, and lungs gradually developed instead of gills. To protect the lungs from mud, a closing valve was evolved. This was the origin of the larynx, which was concerned with respiration and not with the voice. Voice production developed incidentally, as the valve was used to retain air that had been inspired. To illustrate this, think of a frog suddenly disturbed on the bank of a pond. It gulps a supply of air with a snapping sound as it plunges into the water. The sound is not made when the frog enters the water without alarm or hurry — it is made partly by the closing of its mouth, partly by the closing of the valve-like orifice to its lungs. Through the ages, the simple form of larynx possessed by the lower vertebrates has evolved into a marvellous mechanism with many functions, culminating in those of speech and song.

The human larynx is made up of a more or less rigid framework of cartilages held together by ligaments and moved one on another by muscles. It is a box-like structure, approximately 38 mm in length, 32 mm in breadth and 25 mm in depth. It is lined with mucous membrane continuous with that of the pharynx above and of the trachea below. The larynx is separated from the fourth, fifth and sixth cervical vertebrae by the laryngeal portion of the pharynx, the anterior wall of which it forms. In this wall, on each side of the larynx, is a recess known as the piriform fossa. The position of the larynx can be readily seen and felt in the front of the neck where it makes a variable protrusion — 'Adam's apple' or the laryngeal prominence.

Laryngeal cartilages

The chief cartilages of the larynx are: the 'shield-like' *thyroid cartilage* at the front and sides; the 'signet ring' *cricoid cartilage*, whose 'ring' portion lies below the thyroid and whose 'signet' closes the larynx behind; and the right and left *arytenoid cartilages*, which are perched on the 'signet'. The relationship of these cartilages with each other is shown in Figs . 18.1 and 18.2: they articulate by small synovial joints.

In addition to the above cartilages, the *epiglottis* is important. It shares in the protective function of the larynx by covering the

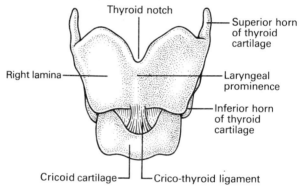

Fig. 18.1. *The thyroid and cricoid cartilages* (*anterior view*).

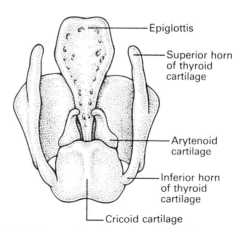

Fig. 18.2. *The laryngeal cartilages* (*posterior view*).

entrance to the larynx during the act of swallowing. The epiglottis is a leaf-shaped portion of cartilage, its stem attached to the posterior aspect of the thyroid cartilage at the junction of the two thyroid plates. It curves upwards behind the tongue and the hyoid bone and cannot move forwards. Small muscles from the arytenoid cartilages pass to the sides of the epiglottis. In swallowing, the arytenoid cartilages are pulled forward, the tongue presses the epiglottis over the narrowed orifice of the larynx, and food slides over the smooth mucous membrane into the oesophagus.

The cartilages of the larynx are attached to each other by sheets and bands of fibrous tissue, containing many elastic fibres. The upper horns of the thyroid cartilage articulate indirectly with the hyoid bone. From this the larynx is suspended. The hyoid bone itself is slung from the jaw by thick muscle, and the tongue is attached to the posterior aspect of the hyoid. Other muscles attach the hyoid bone to the larynx.

Vocal cords

Across the cavity of the larynx, on either side, are folds of tissue called the vocal cords. There are two pairs of these, one called the superior or false cords, and the other called the true vocal cords. The false cords are protective folds of connective tissue passing from half-way up the anterior border of the arytenoid cartilages forward to reach the angle of union between the two laminae of the thyroid cartilage. The true cords pass from the bases of the arytenoid cartilages to points just below the false cords. They are composed of elastic tissue and project further into the cavity of the larynx than do the false cords. The word 'glottis' means the true vocal cords and the space between them (the sound-producing structures). The space depends upon the position of the arytenoid cartilages.

When at rest, the vocal cords are in the V position shown in Fig. 18.3A and no sound is produced. In deep breathing the cords are pulled apart as in Fig. 18.3B. In phonation the cords are adducted, the space between them narrows and in full adduction becomes a mere chink. The muscles which swing the arytenoids out sideways are of the voluntary striated type, so the tension on the cords can be varied at will. The shorter the cords, the more rapid is their vibration as air passes through the glottis, and the higher is the pitch. In producing a 'falsetto' voice, the glottis is much narrowed, as shown

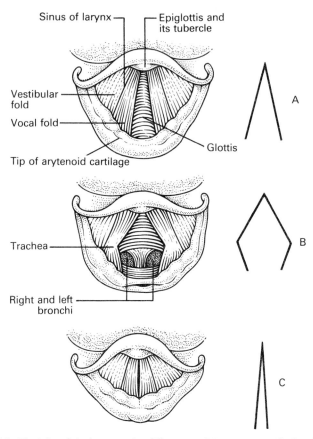

Fig. 18.3. *The inlet of the larynx under different conditions as seen with the aid of a laryngoscope. A. Ordinary quiet inspiration. B. Very deep inspiration. C. Vocalization, especially in singing high notes.*

in Fig. 18.3C. During speech the cords are parallel to each other. The male larynx is larger than the female — the vocal cords are longer and this makes a man's voice deeper. The 'breaking' of a boy's voice at puberty is due to growth changes in the larynx.

Nerves

The nerve supply of the larynx is from:

   1. The superior laryngeal branch of the vagus nerve, with external

and internal branches. The internal branch pierces the thyro-hyoid membrane and passes to the mucous membrane above the level of the cords. The external branch supplies the crico-thyroid muscle only.

2. The recurrent, or inferior laryngeal branch of the vagus nerve, passing to the other intrinsic muscles of the larynx.

Blood vessels

The arteries to the larynx are the superior laryngeal artery, from the external carotid artery, and the inferior laryngeal artery, from a branch of the subclavian artery.

The veins from the larynx enter either the internal jugular vein or the left innominate vein.

Swallowing

The act of swallowing takes place in two stages. First the food bolus is pushed by the tongue into the pharynx, whilst the nasopharynx is shut off by the lifting of the soft palate and the contraction of the superior constrictor muscles of the pharynx. Then the larynx is pulled forcibly upwards and forwards. At this moment, the bolus of food passes backwards over the larynx into the oesophagus, which opens reflexly to receive it.

The portion of the pharynx which lies behind the larynx is normally closed, as the posterior wall of the larynx is closely applied to the vertebral column. The oesophagus is a thin-walled tube commencing at the level of the cricoid cartilage. It passes first downwards, backwards and slightly to the left, then behind the arch of the aorta and the left bronchus, then slightly forwards and left to the opening in the diaphragm (see Fig. 18.4). The lumen of the oesophagus shows 5 constrictions:

1. At its commencement, opposite the sixth cervical vertebra.
2. At the entrance to the thorax.
3. Where the aorta crosses it, opposite the fourth dorsal vertebra.
4. Where the left bronchus crosses it, opposite the fifth dorsal vertebra.
5. Where it passes through the diaphragm, opposite the tenth dorsal vertebra.

Normally, the food is forced by active peristalsis down the oesophagus as far as the diaphragmatic constriction, where its level usually rises and falls once or twice before it passes into the stomach. This is shown by X-ray examination before a fluorescent screen, the patient being given barium emulsion to swallow.

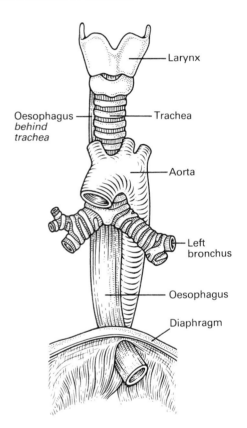

Fig. 18.4. *The relations of the oesophagus.*

19   Diseases of the larynx

Hoarseness is the chief symptom of disease of the larynx. It is the rough grating quality of voice, with a lower pitch than is normal for the individual, due to impaired vibration of the cords in response to the air column in the trachea. Very many diseases give rise to hoarseness, and though it is common with a severe cold or cough, any persistent hoarseness should be investigated, as it is frequently an early sign of serious disease.

Stridor is a harsh shrill sound occurring during respiration when there is partial obstruction of the larynx. In quiet breathing the vocal cords scarcely move, but when obstructed, they are moved forcibly up and down with respiration.

Acute infectious laryngitis in adults

This may occur as an entity but is usually associated with upper respiratory infection. The larynx becomes red and roughened, with, at first, scanty secretion.

Symptoms. These are hoarseness, which ranges from frequent breaking when speaking is attempted to complete loss of voice, a paroxysmal ineffective cough, and aching pain in the larynx. The temperature may rise to about 38°C (100°F) for one or two days.

Complications. In an adult, these are generally comparatively slight. Spread of inflammation, for example, into the trachea is not uncommon and pulmonary complications may follow if the laryngitis is not properly treated.

Treatment. The voice should be rested and steam inhalations given. The accompanying general respiratory infection should be treated.
   Laryngitis occurs as a complication of many acute specific diseases, such as measles, scarlet fever, whooping cough, typhoid fever, and influenza, and in such cases the patient is severely ill. Meanwhile, the larynx and throat are watched so that a low

tracheostomy can be performed should there be signs of obstructive laryngeal dyspnoea.

Acute laryngitis in children (or croup)

The larynx of a child is small in proportion to the development of other regions; and the submucous tissue is looser than in adult life. Therefore, laryngitis in childhood is liable to be a much more serious condition than that described above. Oedema of the tissues and narrowing of the glottis is liable to occur, so dyspnoea may follow in a very short space of time. The condition is sometimes called spasmodic laryngitis. The spasms are short in duration and may be relieved by hot applications over the larynx. Very rarely, the obstruction requires tracheostomy, and instruments for this purpose should be kept in readiness.

Oedematous laryngitis occurs in a number of conditions, both traumatic and infective, and is described in greater detail later in this chapter.

Acute laryngo-tracheo-bronchitis in children

This is a serious condition occurring during epidemics of respiratory diseases and thought to be due to a filter-passing virus. Its onset is sudden and it may show itself as a fulminating laryngitis. Secondary bacterial infection occurs rapidly, particularly with *Haemophilus influenzae*. Not only do the larynx and air passages become swollen, but the thick secretions formed readily cause obstruction and may even produce crusts.

Treatment. This is urgent and consists of giving the child massive doses of an antibiotic, and putting him into a Croupaire tent or steam tent filled with tyloxapol (Alevaire). Tyloxapol is a non-irritating, non-toxic detergent, and its use favours the liquefying of the thick, tenacious secretions.

The child is watched with great care. If the obstruction to the airway increases and the general condition deteriorates, a tracheostomy is needed. The nurse has a special responsibility in such cases and must report instantly any increased restlessness or rise in pulse rate. Tracheostomy should be undertaken before any chest recession or cyanosis occurs.

After a tracheostomy has been carried out, repeated broncho-scopy and suction may be needed in order to free the lower airways of secretions and crusts.

Diphtheria of the larynx

Pharyngeal and nasal diphtheria were considered in earlier sections.

Laryngeal diphtheria (uncommon now, since the discovery of the use of antitoxin) is usually an extension of the disease in the pharynx, but may occur primarily in the larynx, especially in children. The attack may be severe, as the diagnosis is not made as early as in faucial diphtheria and therefore the injection of antitoxin is delayed.

Symptoms. The disease processes are similar to those of pharyngeal diphtheria, but the loose submucous tissue of the larynx swells early, and causes a cough and spasmodic stridor — commonly called 'croup'. The stridor and dyspnoea become increasingly severe. The special odour of the breath and the systemic signs of the disease are the same as in other forms of diphtheria. The diagnosis is usually made by indirect laryngoscopy. In appearance, the larynx is red and swollen; later, patches of grey exudate with slight bleeding at the edges may be seen, and still later a diphtheritic membrane.

Treatment. Antitoxin is given without waiting for confirmation of the diagnosis from culture of the swab. To relieve obstructive dyspnoea, tracheostomy may be required. The general treatment of the disease is as described earlier.

Nocturnal dyspnoea in children

Attacks of dyspnoea at night are frequently causes of great alarm. They occur after a child has been asleep for an hour or more. The dyspnoea is inspiratory, and accompanied by stridor. It lasts for a short period, then normal breathing returns, often with vomiting of thick mucus. The causes may be: (*a*) inflammatory, for example influenza or the onset of diphtheria; (*b*) non-inflammatory, which may be physiological.

Non-inflammatory nocturnal dyspnoea

During sleep, mucous secretions which normally drain from the pharynx into the oesophagus occasionally overflow into the larynx. This causes a sharp cough reflex and the glottis snaps shut, giving rise to air hunger. An attempt at inspiration draws the secretions below the larynx. Violent coughing then expels the residual air, which causes further air hunger. By this time the child is thoroughly awake and frightened. Soon, however, the glottis opens in response to the pull of the laryngeal muscles, the intruding matter is expelled and the coughing subsides with a hoarse croak. The child falls asleep and is quite well in the morning.

Many children have an occasional attack of this kind. If there is enlargement of the tonsils and adenoids, the attacks are more frequent and severe, owing to the increase of secretion and the diminished airway.

Stridor of the newborn

This condition is thought to be due to muscular weakness or incoordination. The entrance to the larynx tends to collapse inwards during inspiration. The stridor may be relieved by putting the infant in the prone position, whilst keeping watch that the nose and mouth are not obstructed. The condition usually settles itself after a few months.

Laryngismus stridulus

This is a condition of childhood, particularly between two and six years of age. It is usually associated with rickets and is due to a lack of Vitamin D.

Symptoms. Without previous symptoms, the child wakens after a few hours' sleep with a peculiar, hollow cough. The cough is quickly followed by a crowing inspiration, and then the typical inspiratory, obstructive laryngeal dyspnoea sets in. The child becomes cyanosed and staring in the struggle for air. Gradually the cough and distress lessens, the attack subsides after one or two hours and the child falls asleep.

Treatment. Reassurance is important. The child should be supported gently, patted and soothed in an encouraging manner. If available, oxygen is the best treatment for the attack. The room air should be kept warm and moist. A steam kettle may be used. The general health should be attended to, and the diet should contain sufficient milk, fruit, and additional vitamins. Artificial sunlight is valuable.

The outlook is good as long as the lack of vitamin D is not allowed to recur.

Angioneurotic oedema

This condition is one form of giant urticaria in which the subcutaneous tissues are involved as well as the skin. It is due to allergy, and there is a nervous system element in the vasomotor disturbances manifested. The oedema may develop rapidly in the course of a few minutes. It affects the eyelids, lips, tongue and throat, causing an alarming sense of suffocation.

Symptoms. A tickling sensation is followed quickly by dyspnoea and signs of obstruction. The voice is muffled and deep. The larynx is so swollen that when viewed in a laryngeal mirror, it appears as a shapeless, purplish mass. Diagnosis is usually easy because of the associated skin condition, or because the patient is known to have suffered from previous attacks.

Treatment. Slow subcutaneous injection of 0.2–0.6 ml of adrenaline hydrochloride will usually relieve the condition. Tracheostomy is rarely necessary, but a sterile set of instruments should be ready.

Local treatment of the larynx is not advised.

Investigation of the cause should be made. Patients subject to angioneurotic oedema should be taught to give themselves adrenaline, as required.

Chronic laryngitis

The causes of persistent inflammation of the larynx are many;

1. Repeated infections of the respiratory tract and damage caused by coughing.

2. Vocal abuse, e.g. too much shouting at sporting events, straining the voice in singing, or using the voice during an acute attack of laryngitis.
3. Constant exposure to dust, tobacco or other smoke and irritants.
4. Mouth breathing.
5. Systemic causes such as alcoholism, which produces chronic vasodilation.
6. Tumours, benign and malignant.
7. Syphilis.
8. Tuberculosis of the larynx, which is always secondary to pulmonary tuberculosis.

Signs. Indirect laryngoscopy shows a patchy, rough redness of the mucosa, which elsewhere is dull pink or grey. A stringy secretion covers the cords. By direct laryngoscopy, the roughness of the mucous membrane is more conspicuous, and the vocal cords appear rounded and thickened. The voice is intermittently hoarse and rough, and the individual is constantly clearing his throat, especially before speech. Chronic laryngitis is so common that this 'ahem' has become a common practice to attract attention at the beginning of a speech.

Symptoms. The patient complains of hoarseness, particularly after a night's sleep or after using the voice all day. The throat aches and feels swollen. A tickling sensation causes a constant slight cough.

Before a diagnosis of 'chronic laryngitis' is made, the possibility of tuberculosis, syphilis, or a new growth must be excluded, generally by biopsy.

Treatment. Search must be made for a focus of infection. This may be in the nose, the sinuses, the tonsils or the teeth. Other predisposing causes, such as smoking, alcohol and dust should be eliminated. Local treatment is not very satisfactory apart from thorough oral hygiene. The patient should be advised to sleep on his side, using a low pillow. This prevents the pharyngeal secretions from trickling into the larynx. Change to a warm moist seaside climate is helpful and a change of occupation must often be seriously considered. Silence is the best treatment, and if this is observed, perfect recovery can occur.

Vocal nodules

These are due to overworking the voice, particularly if inflammation is present. They appear as little white points on the edge of the vocal cords, always at the junction of the anterior with middle third, where the cords hit each other in phonation. With rest, they disappear; otherwise, they enlarge and may reach the size of a small pea.

Symptoms. These are hoarseness, and periodic complete loss of voice, which results from the dropping of the nodule below the cords, where it may be nipped.

Treatment. For the smallest nodules the only treatment is rest of the voice. A large nodule, or one that is not resolving, is removed with punch forceps.

Laryngeal polypi

With hypertrophy of the mucous membrane of the larynx, a polypus may form; there is usually only one. The commonest attachment is to the under surface of the anterior portion of one cord, from which it hangs in the subglottic space. It may not be seen on examination unless the patient is told to cough, when it is blown up and appears above the cords.

Symptoms. Periodic sudden loss of voice occurs with as sudden a return.

Treatment. This is removal by punch forceps or snare under direct vision.

Tuberculosis of the larynx

The larynx is never the seat of primary tuberculosis, but is always secondary to pulmonary tuberculosis. As the latter is becoming rarer, so tuberculosis of the larynx is now very uncommon.

Symptoms. At first the only symptom of a tuberculous larynx is in the voice, which is weak and intermittently husky. Talking is painful. Later, the swelling, ulceration and perichondritis of the arytenoid cartilage leads to fixation of the cricoarytenoid joint and the vocal cord. The voice becomes weaker and more husky, and there is difficulty in swallowing, stridor, cough with sputum, and pain (frequently extending to the ear). Dyspnoea is rare. The outlook depends upon the condition of the lungs.

Signs. Lesions of varying activity may be seen, often on the posterior laryngeal wall, or the interarytenoid region and involving the cords. The ulcers are shallow and indolent. Later, nodules of granulation give an uneven 'mouse-nibbled' appearance to the cords.

Treatment. By the use of streptomycin and PAS, complete healing may be expected. From the nurse's point of view, the treatment is that of open tuberculosis, and she must take the appropriate personal precautions.

Syphilis of the larynx

Primary syphilis does not attack the larynx, but most patients with *secondary syphilis* have some laryngeal involvement. There is some erythema and the vocal cords have a mottled appearance. Occasionally, 'snail-track' ulcers are seen on the epiglottis or arytenoids. The only symptoms are hoarseness and a raw sensation, and the only local treatment is steam inhalations.

Tertiary syphilis often has serious effects:

1. Gummata occur on the epiglottis, arytenoid eminences and false cords. They are deep red or purple, sometimes with a central yellow spot showing an area of softening.
2. Deep ulcers supervene on the gummata. The ulcer has a sharp punched-out edge, with a grey and sloughing base, and is surrounded by an area of congestion.
3. Gummatous perichondritis, chiefly of the thyroid cartilage leads to swelling inside the glottis.
4. During healing the larynx becomes distorted by scar tissue. There may be destruction of the epiglottis, union of the vocal cords, stenosis of the subglottis, and ankylosis of the cricoarytenoid joint.

Symptoms. These correspond to the pathological condition. The patient has a harsh, raucous voice. Extensive ulceration may exist without pain or difficulty in swallowing. Stenosis leads to stridor and dyspnoea which is worse at night, but is so insidious at onset that the patient becomes accustomed to it.

In diagnosis, tuberculosis and malignant disease must be excluded. As the Wassermann and Meinicke reactions are sometimes negative in syphilis of the larynx, a section of a doubtful ulcer is examined under a microscope.

Treatment. Systemic injections of penicillin or of bismuth are given. Permanent tracheostomy may be necessary for stenosis but it must be a low incision, owing to the danger of contraction of scar tissue.

Paralysis of the larynx

The muscles of the larynx are supplied by the recurrent laryngeal nerve. This nerve may be paralysed owing to:

1. Central lesions in the brain stem, as in bulbar palsy and some cerebellar tumours.
2. Lesions affecting the vagus nerve in the neck.
3. Lesions affecting the nerve after it leaves the vagus.

The latter include:

(a) Pressure caused by aortic aneurysm.
(b) Pressure from carcinoma of the bronchus, oesophagus, enlarged thyroid or other glands.
(c) Injury such as cut throat or during operation on the thyroid gland.
(d) Toxic effects of diphtheria, influenza, typhoid fever, syphilis.

The muscles first and most often affected are the abductors of the vocal cords. Paralysis of the adductors is more often hysterical in origin. According to the degree of paralysis, whether unilateral or bilateral, partial or complete, so the symptoms vary.

Sensory paralysis arises from interference with the superior laryngeal nerve. It may be due to pressure or to toxic peripheral neuritis, as in general paralysis of the insane and tabes dorsalis.

The symptoms are anaesthesia, resulting in choking fits due to food going 'the wrong way'.

Treatment. Very often no treatment is necessary, as the larynx learns to compensate for its own deficiency. The cause of the paralysis is treated if possible. Tracheostomy or intubation may be necessary in bilateral paralysis, or a plastic operation on the larynx may be performed. Frequent laryngoscopic aspiration may be used for patients with tabes dorsalis.

Injuries of the larynx

Cut throat

If the larynx is opened in a cut throat, the inhalation of blood will probably produce pulmonary complications. Tracheostomy should be performed below the injury, the latter being packed, and if necessary, repaired.

Blow on the larynx

This may cause fracture of the cartilage or extravasation of blood into the laryngeal tissues. Perichondritis occurs, and fixation of one or both vocal cords, which may become permanent.

Symptoms. There is tenderness over one or more cartilage. Swelling of the perichondrium enlarges the outline of the larynx and may lead to obstruction. Blood-stained sputum may be expectorated, or blood may be seen in the larynx.

Treatment. Unless urgent symptoms appear, no interference is required, but the patient should be kept under observation. If there is much haemorrhage, it may be necessary to open the larynx and tie the bleeding point; obstruction may call for tracheostomy.

Acute obstruction of the larynx

Signs. Laryngeal obstruction of sudden onset or rapid progress needs little diagnosis — the trouble is obvious to any onlooker. The patient, so often a child, is brought to hospital with extreme difficulty of inspiration, accompanied by stridor and an ashy-grey face. Adults may have a grey or bluish tinge to their pallor. The difficulty of breathing is practically always inspiratory for various mechanical reasons and is accompanied by an indrawing of the chest wall. Children are usually very restless from anoxaemia, and this restlessness results in fatigue and desire for sleep. Should the obstruction not be relieved, the child eventually becomes unconscious as respiration ceases. Death from asphyxia can be prevented if the patient comes under surgical care before the heart has ceased to beat. It usually ceases within three or four minutes after cessation of respiration.

The *causes* of laryngeal obstruction are trauma, foreign bodies and disease. The history may make diagnosis obvious. Enquiry should be made as to whether any toy or small object has disappeared. The severity of the *symptoms* of obstruction depends upon the rapidity of its onset. A patient with a slowly developing stenosis of the larynx will learn to breathe slowly and with the least possible exertion, whereas one with a sudden obstruction, frightened at the sense of suffocation, makes violent efforts to take in more air and these close the larynx. The more sudden and violent the inrush of air, the more quickly and tightly do the folds of the glottis close.

The first aid treatment consists in calmly convincing the patient, if an older child or an adult and not unconscious, that he can get more air if he does not try so hard to breathe in, and then in removing the obstruction if possible.

Immediate laryngostomy or tracheostomy may be necessary to save life. The exact cause of the obstruction can be sought and treated later.

Foreign bodies in the larynx

If the obstruction is a foreign body that can be seen, it can sometimes be hooked out with a finger, or removed by forceps. A small child can be picked up by the ankles and thumped on the back.

A large object impacted in the larynx is likely to cause acute obstruction, necessitating immediate tracheotomy. This operation may also be required to relieve the dyspnoea caused by small foreign bodies. Pins, nails and other sharp objects cause sudden pain, cough, loss of voice, and in some cases, spasm of the vocal cords to such a degree that tracheostomy is essential to enable respiration until the foreign body is removed. The spasm usually passes off if the body becomes impacted, but its movements excite fresh attacks and, sometimes, haemoptysis. If the object is not soon removed, inflammatory oedema and abscess may follow, though several years may pass without the development of serious symptoms.

Examination by indirect (with a mirror) or direct laryngoscopy will usually establish the diagnosis. In some cases X-rays may be required. Removal is achieved by straight forceps passed down the tube of a direct laryngoscope.

Benign tumours of the larynx

Innocent new growths of the larynx are comparatively common. Those that occur are papilloma, fibroma and, more rarely, lipoma and angioma.

Papilloma

The growths are usually multiple in children. They are warty, usually pedunculated and may be white, pink or red. They appear to rest on the cords, but may grow from below and on the trachea.

Symptoms. The symptoms are hoarseness only, unless the papillomata are multiple or very large, and then dyspnoea and stridor may occur.

Rapid occurrence often needs tracheostomy.

Fibroma

A fibroma is usually situated on the upper surface of the vocal cord. Such a growth always occurs singly.

Angioma

An angioma presents itself on the cords or the mucous membrane near them. It occasionally gives rise to haemoptysis.

Treatment of fibromas and angiomas. This consists of removal by laryngeal forceps passed under direct vision through a laryngoscope. Both tumours are usually small and easily nipped off, but the latter may need the application of a cautery to check haemorrhage and this should be followed by laryngofissure — the surgical splitting of the thyroid cartilage — in order to remove the growth.

Malignant tumours of the larynx

These are relatively uncommon, but occur ten times more often in men than in women. This may be due to better oral hygiene and less abuse of the voice by women. They usually affect the middle-aged or elderly, and are of the squamous-celled carcinoma type. Metastatic deposits in the larynx are rare, and laryngeal growths themselves seldom metastasize. The growths are classified as:

1. *Intrinsic tumours* — inside the larynx. These generally arise from the vocal cords and grow slowly.
2. *Extrinsic tumours.* These mostly commence outside the larynx and therefore are more accurately classified as pharyngeal tumours. They may develop on the epiglottis, the aryepiglottic folds or the piriform fossa. Their growth is more rapid and involves the lymphatics early. They are therefore more difficult to treat and are much more serious than intrinsic tumours.

Intrinsic tumours

Symptoms. At first, hoarseness is the only symptom. Later, when the growth spreads to the opposite cord, there is pain, cough and dyspnoea. Still later, the voice becomes a whisper, and the growth becomes extrinsic.

Extrinsic tumours

Symptoms. These are discomfort and, later, pain on swallowing, sore throat, and painful ear. Symptoms are often vague and intermittent. A node may present itself first. The voice is affected only if the growth spreads to the glottis. It causes increasing difficulty and pain on swallowing. A patient with an extrinsic malignant tumour of the larynx exhibits marked signs of cachexia.

To make a correct diagnosis of the laryngeal tumour, it is frequently necessary to remove a section for examination by microscope.

Treatment of intrinsic and extrinsic laryngeal tumours

Intrinsic tumours. Early growths limited to one cord are treated by either radiation or implantation of radium needles. Advanced growths usually require a total laryngectomy. If glands are present, these are removed at the same time.

Extrinsic tumours. The treatment of these growths is by radiotherapy, with the lymphatic glands being removed by surgery. The postoperative nursing care here is extremely important.

Sometimes no curative treatment is possible, owing to the advanced stage of the disease or the age and weakness of the patient, and sometimes the treatment attempted is unsuccessful. Even so, good nursing can help to cheer the patient considerably and reduce his discomfort.

Complications and their treatment. The complications which eventually terminate life are dysphagia, asphyxia, haemorrhage and sepsis. For the increasing dysphagia, gastrostomy is sometimes performed. Should there be sudden dyspnoea and respiratory obstruction, a low tracheostomy may be required, but as a rule the obstruction comes on so gradually that the patient, who is usually in bed, is not distressed by it.

The teeth and mouth must be kept as clean as possible. Once the tumour begins to ulcerate, the mouth becomes very septic, the breath has a sickly odour, abscesses occur, and the cervical glands are enlarged and tender. Septic absorption causes rapid wasting and loss of strength. Alkaline cleansing lotions are used for the mouth, and frequent mouthwashes should be given. Antiseptic and deodorant throat lozenges are also helpful and are best sucked after meals.

Small amounts of liquid paraffin may be given two or three times a day, as straining from constipation must be avoided.

In the later stages of the growth, neuralgic pain is marked. Aspirin mixtures may relieve this at first, but morphine becomes necessary in increasing doses and helps to relieve distress from other causes.

20 Operations on the larynx and pharynx

Tracheostomy

The term 'tracheotomy' strictly means an opening into the trachea. 'Tracheostomy' is the correct term for an opening which is to be kept patent.

The operation, by making an opening through the neck into the trachea, provides an airway in cases of impending asphyxia due to laryngeal obstruction. It has recently been performed increasingly for other kinds of respiratory difficulty — e.g. in paralysis, head injuries, tetanus, chronic bronchitis, bronchopneumonia, etc. The object is not only to provide assisted respiration by intermittent positive pressure, but also to aspirate secretions and prevent aspiration into the lungs. In these cases a cuffed tracheostomy tube is used (see Fig. 20.1). This is made of disposable polythene. The operation may be one of two types: planned or emergency.

Planned tracheostomy

In the great majority of cases tracheostomy is performed under local anaesthesia, as any patient requiring the operation will be liable to respiratory difficulty with a general anaesthetic, unless he can be intubated. The patient should be reassured, told that the operation

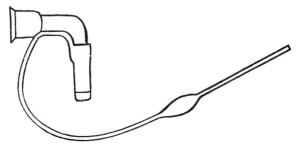

Fig. 20.1. *Cuffed Radcliffe tracheostomy tube.*

will only take a few minutes, that he will feel no pain and very little discomfort. The skin of the neck, from the tip of the chin to half-way down the sternum should be shaved, washed, and prepared according to the customary requirements of the surgeon.

The instruments for tracheostomy are:

1. Tracheostomy tubes. There is widespread use of disposable tubes with wide bore and no inner tube, but non-disposable ones, e.g. Durham's tube, are still used. These consist of:
   (a) Outer tube.
   (b) Inner tube.
   (c) Pilot.
   (d) Tapes looped to the fittings on the outer tube, one end short and one long enough to come round the neck and tie at one side. The tube or cannula must be long enough to reach into the lumen of the trachea from the skin surface. The flanges are adjustable on the outer end of the tubes for this purpose. As long a tube as possible is used. The usual sizes are: Number 5 for an adult, 4 for an adolescent, 2 or 3 for children and 1 for infants.
2. Scalpels or small Bard–Parker's knife with blades.
3. Two small, blunt hook retractors.
4. A sharp hook.
5. Tracheal dilators, e.g. Bowlby's.
6. Six pairs of small artery forceps.
7. Pointed dissecting scissors.
8. Small, full-curved suture needles.
9. Full-curved skin needles.
10. Needle holder.
11. Suture material.
12. Ligatures, e.g. steel, silk, nylon.
13. Hypodermic syringe for the local anaesthetic, with reinforced bent needles.
14. Gauze swabs with X-ray opaque marker.
15. Disposable catheters for aspiration through the tracheal tube.
16. Suction apparatus, preferably electric.

Cylinders of, or piped, oxygen should be at hand, and also the bronchoscopic outfit in case of necessity.

The patient lies on his back and his shoulders may be slightly raised on pillows on the operating table. A child should be pinned in a blanket. A sand-bag is placed under the shoulders so as to extend the head, which must be held exactly in the midline by an assistant.

The skin having been prepared, the local anaesthetic is injected into the tissues from the level of the hyoid bone to the suprasternal notch. An incision is then made through the skin and superficial fascia transversely over the thyroid isthmus. Any bleeding vessels are clamped and the incision is then deepened to the cricoid cartilage and the tracheal rings. The isthmus of the thyroid gland may be retracted out of the way, or it may be clamped, divided and ligatured, which is the usual preference. The wound is then thoroughly dried by mopping with gauze swabs, and the trachea is fixed with the sharp hook or tenaculum forceps and is incised in the midline through the third, fourth and fifth rings. Great care is taken not to cut the membranous wall at the back of the trachea. As soon as the trachea is opened, there is a hiss of air and sometimes a little spluttering, but the edges of the wound usually close quickly. The tracheal dilators are therefore immediately inserted. Any clot of mucus present may be coughed out at this point, and if dyspnoea has been at all severe, the patient gives a deep sign of relief. Frequently, an exhausted child has fallen asleep on the operating table.

The surgeon usually then trims the edges of the incision to make an oval opening through which the cannula is inserted. If the cannula is of the proper length, the shield will stand out a little from the level of the skin. The pilot is removed and the tapes are tied lightly round the neck. The wound is closed with interrupted sutures, not too close to the tube. The nurse can then release the patient's head. A dressing is applied, of about six layers of folded gauze, cut halfway down, so as to fit round the tube under the shields.

After-care. A well-ventilated room is prepared for the reception of the patient from theatre. The patient is placed in bed, in a semi-recumbent or sitting position, unless this is contraindicated by his general condition. He must be visible to the nursing staff at all times.

The following apparatus should be available on a trolley beside the patient:

1. A spare tracheostomy tube of the correct size.
2. A pair of tracheal dilators.
3. Fine disposable catheters, size 12.

4. A bowl with a solution for sucking through the catheter and suction tubing.
5. Gauze swabs.
6. Disposable gloves.
7. A large paper bag for all used materials.

Oxygen and suction apparatus should be available within the bed area. Materials for the cleaning and moistening of the mouth must also be to hand.

The special duty of the nurse is to see that the airway is kept clear. Any secretion that is coughed out through the tube should be quickly but gently wiped away, so that it is not sucked back into the trachea. Suction should be applied whenever there is secretion to be aspirated. Rattling or bubbling noises in the patient's respiration show that the secretions are blocking the tube. To apply suction, the catheter is passed down the tracheostomy tube for 25–50 mm. The suction apparatus is then switched on, and the catheter is slowly removed with gentle rotation. The catheter and tubing are then sucked through with the cleansing material. This cleans the suction tubing, and the catheter is disposed of into the bag. When non-disposable tubes are used, the nurse should remove the inner tube at least every hour for the first few days, and replace it with another sterilized tube. To remove it, she should steady the outer tube by pressing it against the neck with her fingers.

The outer tube is changed — on the first occasion by the surgeon, and thereafter by competent nursing staff. This is done within 36 hours of the operation, to remove blood clots and secretions. Afterwards, changing every two or three days is sufficient. The nurse should change the dressings as often as they become soiled. Should the outer tube become dislodged, no time should be lost in replacing it with the duplicate tube which is kept in readiness. In the meantime the nurse should maintain the airway by inserting the tracheal dilators. The dilators are inserted from the side with the blades closed, and the handles are then brought round to the midline and gently opened.

As there is no post-anaesthetic vomiting to be feared, the patient is able and should be encouraged to begin swallowing liquids at any time. Liquids should be given liberally and there is seldom any need for a feeding tube. Any leakage through the tube should of course be reported at once.

The nurse must realize that the patient is voiceless — he cannot call for help; a baby cannot cry aloud. Preprinted, illustrated communication cards indicating the patient's needs are especially useful for children. A firm writing pad and pencil may be provided for the adult patient, together with a bell, which should always be within easy reach. The patient may be anxious and distressed at his inability to speak aloud. He should be reassured that this is only because air leaks through the tube, and that he will be able to talk well after some days by putting his finger over the opening of the tube.

Rest is important, and the patient should be disturbed as little as possible. On the other hand, he should move about early and may usually sit out of bed, should his general condition allow this, on the first postoperative day. The skin sutures are removed on the sixth day. After this, the sterile dressings around the tube are unnecessary. The patient is encouraged to breathe deeply and to cough, being supplied with gauze swabs or paper handkerchiefs to catch mucus. The majority of patients requiring a permanent tracheostomy are fitted with a plastic tracheostomy tube and are taught to manage this themselves. They are then able to go home, instructions being given concerning attendance at the Out-Patients' Department.

Emergency tracheostomy

No one should be allowed to suffocate from absolute laryngeal obstruction for want of a bold attempt at tracheostomy on the part of an onlooker. It may be possible to use the instruments of an already-sterilized tracheostomy set, but if these are not accessible, the operation can be performed with a knife and a dilator (possibly improvised).

The position of the patient and the operation follow the same general lines as for a planned tracheostomy, except that there is no time for the usual skin preparation though there may be time to cleanse quickly with ether, methylated or surgical spirit, and a local anaesthetic is not necessary as the patient is unconscious or nearly so. The fingers of the operator's left hand are used to fix and identify the trachea, and no attempt is made to pick up bleeding points.

The head must be held straight since the incision must be in the midline. The trachea is identified by its ridged structure with the left index finger and is fixed in the midline with the left thumb and middle finger. When the incision has been made, a dilator must be inserted — using artery forceps or the knife handle if necessary — and the incision kept open until a tracheostomy tube can be put in. It may be necessary to apply artificial respiration and give oxygen to re-establish breathing. The severed blood vessels quickly stop bleeding with the fall of the raised pressure due to the asphyxia.

In some cases of asphyxia it may be possible and advisable to insert a bronchoscope, establish regular respiration through it and then perform an orderly tracheostomy. The operation is quite simple if the bronchoscope is in position.

Complications following tracheostomy

Surgical emphysema. If the incision is made too big and air escapes round the tube, surgical emphysema may occur.

If, during the early dressings, the tracheostomy tube is incorrectly replaced, a false passage may be made which will not only cause dyspnoea but will allow air to penetrate the cervical tissue and leak downwards into the mediastinum or upwards to the head. The emphysema produces swelling and a distinctive crackling sound on palpation. Little treatment is required once the tube's position has been corrected. The air is gradually reabsorbed and the discomfort it caused soon passes. As the swelling subsides, the tapes will become loose and should be retied when necessary.

Atelectasis. This complication is often wrongly diagnosed as pneumonia. It is completely relieved by the aspiration of the obstructive plug of mucus, blood clot or tissue by means of a sucker, through a bronchoscope.

Stenosis of the larynx or trachea. Stenosis, if not the cause for which tracheostomy was performed, is most often consequent upon too high a tracheostomy. It may also be due to a badly-fitting cannula or to sepsis.

The tracheostomy should not be above the second ring of the trachea. If a patient is obliged to wear a tracheostomy tube for a long period, it should be checked to see that it fits perfectly. A plastic tube is usually provided for a patient with a permanent opening. If a badly-fitting tube is worn, or if it is not kept clean, there will be erosion of the mucous lining of the trachea, followed by inflammation and necrosis of the cartilage. Stenosis will cause hoarseness and dyspnoea, when attempts are made to remove or occlude the tracheostomy tube.

Pneumothorax. Due to injury of the pleura leading to pulmonary collapse.

Removal of a tracheostomy tube

The process of encouraging the patient to do without his tracheostomy tube is one requiring patience and skill. Since breathing through the nose is not as simple as breathing through the tube, the simple removal of the latter may cause panic especially in a child. First, it is necessary to make sure that breathing through the larynx is possible. The tracheostomy tube worn must be small enough to allow air from the nose to pass round it. Then the tube is partially occluded by a cork cut lengthwise in half. Special rubber corks are used, as ordinary corks are liable to break. When the patient has been able to sleep comfortably for two or three nights with such a cork, it is changed for one that occludes three-quarters of the tube, then for one occluding seven-eights, and finally for one completely closing the tube. The tracheostomy tube is then removed and the patient continues to breathe by the normal route. If the tube has only been worn for a few weeks, the fistula quickly closes, but if it has been worn for several months, stratified epithelium will have grown over the passage and this prevents healing. Very little air leaks out but the mucus which does is most uncomfortable for the patient, and therefore a simple paring and suturing of the wound is carried out. This leaves an almost imperceptible scar.

If the detubation process takes more then one or two weeks, it points to stenosis. The treatment is dilatation, usually achieved by the insertion of rubber or plastic core moulds which are inserted via the larynx with the aid of a special introducer and a laryngoscope.

Laryngostomy

This is a temporary opening for respiration made through the cricothyroid membrane. It is occasionally used instead of tracheostomy, being quicker and less difficult, but it is not so satisfactory. If it becomes necessary to keep a tube for some time in the airway, a tracheostomy is usually performed and the laryngostomy wound allowed to close. Laryngostomy is only suitable for adults.

Local anaesthesia is employed, if time allows. The patient lies supine with his head extended and fixed. A traverse incision 25 mm long is made over the cricothyroid membrane, which is then opened transversely with a narrow knife or sharp-pointed scissors. A flat Butlin's laryngostomy tube or a small tracheostomy tube is then inserted and secured as for tracheostomy.

Laryngectomy and pharyngolaryngectomy

These operations are most often performed for removal of malignant tumour of the larynx — occasionally for the relief of rare forms of laryngeal stenosis. In the treatment of cancer of the larynx or pharynx, the operation chosen depends on the amount of tissue involved. Growths involving the pharynx as well as the larynx are commonly removed by a laryngectomy combined with a partial pharyngectomy.

Preoperative treatment. The preparation of the patient is similar to that for tracheostomy, but since laryngectomy is a much more serious operation and is not an emergency procedure a longer period is devoted to improving the patient's state of nutrition and to oral hygiene. The patient's teeth and gums must be in a healthy state, even if this means postponing the operation for a week or two. His heart, lungs, blood and urine are examined, the blood is grouped and cross-matched, and haemoglobin is estimated. He will be distressed at the thought that he will not be able to talk after the operation, but he can be assured that the structures which form his words will not be affected and that lessons in voice production can be given. These may begin before the operation. The patient is taught to swallow air into the oesophagus and bring it up again noisily, forming the sound into words with his tongue, lips, cheeks and palate.

The patient is admitted several days prior to operation. It is important for him to get to know the ward staff and for them to gain his confidence. It is helpful for him to meet the speech therapist and to know about the postoperative therapy. Meeting a patient who has had a successful laryngectomy is also helpful in enabling him to adjust. The medicosocial worker may need to contact the patient's employer in cases where later redeployment may be necessary.

On the day before operation the patient has his usual diet. Antibiotics are commenced. If the bowels have not been open, a small enema or suppository is given. A sedative is usually needed to ensure a night's sleep. On the morning of operation the face and neck are shaved and the skin cleansed with soap and water. The premedication (e.g. pethidine or morphine and atropine) is given one and a half to one hour prior to operation. Morphine is contraindicated after operation on account of its effect in producing depression of the respiratory centre.

A tracheostomy is performed in the theatre and a blood transfusion is started.

Varieties of operation. The more common operations for the removal of laryngeal or pharyngeal tumours are:

1. Laryngofissure, or median thyrotomy — also known as partial laryngectomy.
2. Total laryngectomy.
3. Pharyngolaryngectomy.

A local anaesthetic is sometimes considered sufficient for all these operations, but fuller anaesthesia may be preferred, such as that produced by the following: cervical block, intravenous thiopentone sodium (Pentothal), or gas, oxygen and ether. If there is respiratory obstruction, a rubber nasal airway may be introduced or an intranasal catheter. Bronchoscopic instruments should be prepared.

Laryngofissure. In this operation the larynx is split down the midline after a preliminary tracheostomy. The growth is removed with parts of one or both vocal cords. The larynx is then closed, the tracheostomy being kept open for approximately 24 hours.

The nursing is similar to that of tracheostomy. For the purpose of taking nourishment, the patient should be told to lean slightly forward and take a good swallow rather than to sip. No talking above a whisper should be allowed for the first few days.

Total laryngectomy. For advanced malignant disease of the larynx, the whole organ is removed. The severed lower part of the trachea is brought up to the skin surface and sewn into position forming a permanent orifice. A laryngectomy tube is inserted into the tracheal orifice after operation. This tube may well be in situ for only two to three weeks.

Postoperative treatment. The nursing requirements are similar to those of tracheostomy, except that this patient will have a nasogastric tube in situ for the first 24–48 hours.

A small amount of blood-stained serous discharge is expected from the orifice over the first 24 hours. This will diminish with time.

The operation of laryngectomy is not usually associated with postoperative shock or pain, and therefore blood transfusion and controlled drugs are rarely prescribed. Many patients will have an intravenous infusion of normal saline and dextrose 5%, to maintain electrolyte balance. Should the patient complain of pain, a mild soluble analgesic may be prescribed for installation into the nasogastric tube.

As soon as the patient's blood pressure and pulse are stable, the patient may be raised to either the semirecumbent, or upright, position in bed.

Feeding is by the nasogastric tube, and most hospital dietetic departments will prepare a fluid nutritious diet to maintain the calorific intake of the patient until he can resume a normal diet. A few hours after operation, the patient will be able to take sips of water to keep his mouth moist. Frequent mouthwashes should also be given to keep the patient's mouth fresh and moist.

The first dressing of the laryngectomy wound is normally performed by the surgeon, after which the task becomes a nursing procedure which is performed daily, or more often if the dressing material becomes moist. Aseptic technique is always used until the sutures are removed, approximately four to six days after operation, depending on the condition of the wound. The laryngectomy tube will be removed permanently two to three weeks after the operation.

The patient is encouraged to get up and dress as soon as possible. Discharge from hospital is at around 14–21 days. An appointment for the Out-Patients' Department is given, and an appointment to commence speech therapy is also arranged. The patient is encouraged to return to work as soon as possible.

Radiotherapy is rarely required postoperatively.

Pharyngolaryngectomy. This may be undertaken as a one-stage operation or a two-stage procedure. After a tracheostomy and a laryngectomy, the growth is removed from the pharynx. Skin flaps taken from the thigh as a donor area are sutured to the edges of the cut pharynx and used to form a channel into the oesophagus. A feeding tube is passed along this channel into the stomach.

Postoperative treatment. The nursing after pharyngolaryngectomy follows the same lines as after laryngectomy. A great deal of saliva at first leaks from the pharyngostomy and therefore dressings need frequent changing. It is most important to clear the oesophageal tube after each feed and to make certain that it is patent before the next feed is given, as the tube cannot be moved during the healing of the graft. After a few days it is usually found that fluid given by mouth will trickle down the pharyngeal gutter and leakage becomes steadily less. The feeding tube can be removed after a week and repositioned in the oesophagus behind the tracheostome. Closure should take place in three weeks; nasal feeding frequently follows for some days after its removal. Oral feeding can be commenced when the graft has taken and healed satisfactorily. Swallowing must be tested first. The tracheostomy is kept open for three or four days after operation. The thigh wound is treated as for a skin graft and is dressed according to the instructions of the surgeon.

Antibiotics and sulphonamides are of inestimable value in minimizing local sepsis. The patient may be ordered Vitamin C, and iron tablets may be crushed and given with feeds.

Secondary closure of the pharyngostomy can be carried out after about three weeks, with plastic reconstruction of the swallowing tube.

21 The inhalation or ingestion of foreign bodies — endoscopy

Of all the emergencies dealt with in an Ear, Nose and Throat Unit, those of the most common occurrence, apart from acute ear conditions, are due to the lodging of a foreign body in the deeper air or food passages. An appalling mortality rate existed until the beginning of this century, since when the development of special methods of diagnosis and treatment has considerably decreased it. These methods are known as *endoscopy*, the use of illuminating instruments which are introduced into the air or food passages in order to show the foreign body and facilitate its removal. The direct, or illuminated laryngoscope has already been referred to. Through it, other instruments such as a bronchoscope or forceps can be passed. An oesophagoscope is used to illuminate and remove objects in the oesophagus.

Generally speaking, foreign bodies impacted in the trachea, bronchi and oesophagus, if not removed, ultimately prove fatal from such causes as lung abscess or mediastinal infection. In almost every case the offending object can be removed through the mouth by endoscopy. Waiting for spontaneous expulsion is dangerous; blind methods of removal are extremely dangerous.

Foreign body in the larynx

This was discussed in Chapter 20.

Foreign body in the trachea

In tracheal obstruction, the spasm of the larynx is much less than that occurring in laryngeal obstruction, but the stridor caused by the dyspnoea accompanies both inspiration and expiration. Should the obstruction be due to an inhaled foreign body, the choking attack which occurs as the object passes through the larynx ceases as it falls into the trachea, but a harsh cough persists and the breathing is laborious. The patient sits forward with the head flexed in an attempt to ease the strain on the trachea. If the foreign body is movable, the cough is paroxysmal. The diagnosis may be confirmed by X-ray or by endoscopy. A longer tube is required than for laryngoscopy. Removal may be made by tracheostomy, should endoscopy not be available.

Foreign body in the bronchus

An inhaled object is a common cause of bronchial obstruction. As foreign bodies may be of all shapes, sizes and consistency, the conditions to which they give rise when lodged in a bronchus vary a great deal. The size of the foreign body in relation to the age of the patient is important, as upon this depends the site of impaction and consequently the area of lung that may be affected. Peas and beans, which have frequently been inhaled by children, swell rapidly, causing acute inflammation and oedema of the mucosa, with consequent dyspnoea. Should there be obstruction of a main bronchus, complete collapse (atelectasis) of that lung may follow. Alternatively, the object may set up a ball-valve action, allowing air to pass it on inspiration, but not on expiration. Emphysema—the presence of air outside the air passages—then occurs. The patient has an asthmatic wheeze and feeling of tightness in the chest. An unsuspected foreign body—perhaps the patient had a choking fit during the inhalation of the object which was then drawn into a smaller bronchus—may give rise to bronchiectasis or lung abscess. Foreign bodies are more likely to be inhaled into the right bronchus than into the left, as the right is more nearly a continuation of the trachea than is the left. It is also slightly larger than the left bronchus.

Once the foreign body has been removed, and bronchoscopic aspiration carried out, it is remarkable how quickly the patient gets well.

Swallowed foreign bodies

Patients frequently come or are brought into hospital with clear histories of having swallowed objects of various shapes and sizes.

The oesophagus has a surprising capacity of distension and cases have been reported in which a complete dental plate has been swallowed during sleep.

Sometimes quite small objects become arrested, and sharp ones can cause much damage. For example, open safety pins with points uppermost, sharp irregular bones or brooches may pierce the oesophageal wall or cause a tear unless they are removed with great care. The great majority of foreign bodies are arrested at the uppermost constriction. In this situation, coins stick transversely.

Foreign body in the oesophagus

Symptoms. There is usually a feeling of something sticking. Should the object be sharp, for example a sharp bone, there is actual pain on swallowing. Occasionally, there is dyspnoea, wheezing or cough due to compression of the air passages from behind or from trickling of secretion into the larynx.

Treatment. An X-ray examination should be carried out before attempting to remove a foreign body, and a barium swallow is sometimes given if a non-opaque object is suspected. When the site of impaction has been ascertained, oesophagoscopy should be undertaken. The nurse should prepare a complete set of broncho-scopic as well as oesophageal tubes and instruments. in case of need. The foreign body having been located through the oeso-phagoscope, it is carefully extracted with suitable forceps.

ENDOSCOPY

Endoscopy is carried out in an operating theatre. There is frequently one attached to the Out-Patients' Department of the Ear, Nose and Throat Unit for such purpose.

The preparation of the patient is similar for all endoscopy of the respiratory and alimentary tracts.

Unless the case is one of extreme urgency, the usual pharyngeal and laryngeal examinations are made, the lungs are tested by auscultation for air entry and the oesophagus for swallowing function.

The patient is given a general or a local anaesthetic, according to the size of the instrument used. For both types of anaesthesia, the stomach should be empty to avoid vomiting. If general anaesthesia is desired, a basal anaesthetic followed by gas and oxygen is most satisfactory. Before local anaesthesia, which is frequently preferred, especially for bronchoscopy as then the patient is able to co-operate with the surgeon, the patient is usually given an injection, such as morphine 16 mg, scopolamine 0.5 mg and atropine 0.6 mg. About 1 ml of 10% solution of cocaine hydrochloride is then sprayed on the fauces and pharynx. A laryngeal applicator is tipped with wool moistened in the cocaine solution and applied to the inner surface of both lips, over the base of the tongue, over the posterior pharyngeal wall, the laryngeal aspect of the epiglottis and so into each piriform fossa where the main sensory nerve runs.

After anaesthesia has been produced, the patient may sit astride a stool and hold his chin forward and head tilted back, but the recumbent position is generally more satisfactory and comfortable. The patient lies on his back on the operating table, with his shoulders as far as the middle of the scapulae projecting over the end. An adjustable head-rest is usually fitted to the table—if not, an assistant supports the head in the same position as described for the seated patient. The head must always be kept exactly in the midline.

Direct laryngoscopy

Various sizes of laryngoscope should be at hand. The nurse should see that a reserve of electric bulbs is available and that the electric connections are in order. Suction apparatus will be needed, as accumulated saliva will trickle down the trachea and cause coughing if not aspirated. Swallowing is almost impossible with the laryngoscope is position. Aspiration is carried out either through a channel in the laryngoscope or through an independent tube. Tracheostomy instruments should be in readiness if a foreign body is to be removed, lest it should be dislodged and fall into the trachea. All instruments used in endoscopy should be sterile. Sterilization in a formalin cabinet is a satisfactory method, especially for the illuminating instruments. They can be stored in the cabinet and should be rinsed in sterile water before use.

By means of the direct laryngoscope, a brilliantly illuminated image of the larynx can be obtained. The spatula end of the instrument is passed over the tongue until the epiglottis is identified. The epiglottis is then lifted forward and the glottis and cords exposed. Beyond these can be seen the trachea, and one or both bronchial orifices. The laryngoscope is usually passed on through the glottis to examine the sub-glottic area and the trachea. It is then slightly withdrawn and passed into the laryngopharynx to show the posterior wall of the larynx. Laryngoscopy may now be carried out through an operating microscope.

Bronchoscopy

For the introduction of a bronchoscope, a laryngoscope with a removable slide is first passed. The bronchoscope is a long slender tube which may be single or have one extension tube telescoping into the other. There are numerous perforations in the distal part of the tube to allow air to pass in and out. A watch spring is fitted to the proximal end of the extension tube. This spring is engraved with a centimetre scale to enable the surgeon to read off the total length of the tube which has been introduced.

The surgeon passes the laryngoscope and holds it with his left hand. The bronchoscope is held in his right hand and passed through the laryngoscope. When the surgeon sees the vocal cords abduct during inspiration, he slips the slanted end of the bronchoscope between the two cords with a slightly rotary motion. The slide which forms part of the barrel of the laryngoscope is pushed up and the laryngoscope removed, leaving the bronchoscope with its end free in the trachea. The tube can then be carefully moved down and rotated in order to obtain different views of the bronchial tree.

Oesophagoscopy

An oesophagoscope is similar to a sigmoidoscope, being a much larger instrument than the bronchoscope. The common type has a drainage canal in order to aspirate secretion without interruption during oesophagoscopy. An oesophageal speculum is necessary, as the lumen of the oesophagus must be located before the oesophagoscope is passed into it. Thereafter, oesophagoscopy resembles bronchoscopy. Local anaesthesia may be supplemented by intravenous thiopentone sodium (Pentothal), particularly if the passage is difficult due to long upper teeth.

Gastroscopy

The stomach may be inspected through an oesophagoscope. Frequently, a flexible gastroscope is used for this purpose.

Precautions. After the throat has been cocainized for direct endoscopy, the cough reflex will be absent for some time. Special precautions must be taken so that the patient does not inhale fluid or food. This will be discussed further in Chapter 23.

Patients with such disorders are frequently admitted to an Ear, Nose and Throat Unit, as the necessary investigations include oesophagoscopy, which is a technique in which the laryngologist specializes.

Oesophageal diseases, apart from impacted foreign bodies, are classified into:

1. Neuromuscular disorders — diverticulitis and achalasia.
2. Strictures from fibrosis — e.g. following burns or peptic ulcers.
3. Strictures from malignant tissue.

Neuromuscular disorders of the oesophagus

Achalasia or cardiospasm

In this condition, the oesophagus gradually, over many years, becomes dilated and hypertrophied and develops an obstruction at its lower end. The cause is unknown but thought to be due to inco-ordination of the autonomic nerve supply. The sufferers are usually women.

Signs. Examination by X-ray after a barium meal will show the lower end of the oesophagus to be dilated, becoming sigmoid in advanced cases. Obstruction at the cardiac sphincter, where the oesophagus enters the stomach, will also be shown.

If an oesophagoscope is passed after suction of the contents of the dilated oesophagus, the mucous membrane will appear inflamed and ulcerated. Malignant change in the ulcers sometimes occurs.

Symptoms. A gradually increasing difficulty of swallowing leads to emaciation. There is an unpleasant odour to the breath, as the dilated oesophagus contains undigested and decomposing food and liquid.

Treatment. The cardiospasm may be relieved by repeated dilatation by means of swallowing a Hurst's bougie, which is a long rubber tube containing mercury. If operative treatment is decided upon, the patient is transferred to a ward for thoracic surgery. In Heller's operation, a thoracic approach is made and the lower end of the oesophagus freed. The muscle fibres are then divided in a manner similar to Rammstedt's operation on the pyloric sphincter.

Pharyngeal pouch

A pressure pouch, often termed an 'oesophageal diverticulum' but being truly a portion of the pharyngeal mucosa and connective tissue, becomes squeezed out between the fibres of the inferior constrictor muscles and sags down behind the oesophagus. The cause is thought to be inco-ordination between the sympathetic and parasympathetic nerve supplies.

Symptoms. The symptoms are dysphagia, caused by the pressure on the back of the oesophagus by the food in the pouch, and regurgitation of the undigested food. The majority of patients are elderly, emaciated men. The condition and symptoms increase gradually. Often a gurgling sound can be obtained by pressure with the fingers on the swelling which appears in the neck after eating.

Diagnosis is made from the distinctive signs and symptoms and by radiography. Oesophagoscopy is usually performed in order to inspect and confirm the condition.

Treatment. The pouch is excised through an opening in the side of the neck. After operation, tube feeding is required for about a week.

Alternatively, the 'spur' between the pouch and the oesophagus can be destroyed by electrocoagulation applied through an endoscope (Dohlman's operation).

Burns of the oesophagus

Burns from swallowing hot liquids are rare, but occasionally corrosives are swallowed by accident or intent and cause chemical burns of the oesophagus. Household ammonia, caustic soda disinfectant solutions, and the sulphuric acid used in accumulators are examples of fluids that are sometimes taken in mistake for water. The corrosive effect is usually, but not always, exerted on the lips, tongue and pharynx, as well as on the oesophagus. Sometimes the fluid passes quickly into the stomach and the burning of the oesophagus is very shallow, but if it lingers in the oesophagus the damage caused is very severe.

The diagnosis is usually made on the evidence of the patient or parents, and by the burns of the mouth. Weeks or months later, scarring leads to stricture formation.

Treatment. The first-aid treatment consists of neutralizing an alkali with weak vinegar, and an acid with magnesia or sodium bicarbonate solution. The patient must be encouraged to drink whichever fluid is required, in spite of pain on swallowing. Demulcents such as milk or beaten egg are given. Sometimes there is an accumulation of saliva in the mouth, as the patient is afraid to swallow. This may be aspirated, and then a little bismuth powder is often sprinkled on the tongue and washed down with water. This should be repeated every half-hour for a few days, less often after that. Water must be given regularly and dehydration avoided. Steroids are given early to lessen fibrosis, and an antibiotic to limit the infection to sloughing.

After about two weeks, very gentle oesophagoscopy is carried out every week or ten days in an attempt to prevent narrowing of the oesophagus by scar tissue, which, however, is a common sequel to burning.

A modern line of treatment is to expose the pharynx by incision in the neck and to create a pharyngostome. A feeding tube of large size is inserted and left in place for perhaps two to three months. Antibiotics and cortisone are given to limit sepsis and scarring.

Non-malignant stenosis of the oesophagus

This is commonly due to swallowing corrosive fluids, but may follow ulceration caused by syphilis or other disease. The stricture is most apt to form at the narrowing caused by the crossing of the left bronchus, but there are frequently other strictures present wherever ulcers heal.

Symptom. The symptom is the regurgitation of food.

Treatment. If the stricture is severe, gastrostomy is necessary, after which, the stricture may be excised and the oesophageal stump anastomosed with the stomach. This operation will be carried out in a department for general or thoracic surgery.

If the stricture is patent, the treatment consists of gradual and repeated dilatation. This is frequently done by passing bougies through an oesophagoscope. Another method is to give the patient a silk thread to swallow. Gastrostomy is performed and the end of the thread is brought out through the incision. On the silk are threaded three graduated metal olives and an endless chain is made. The olives are swallowed, brought out of the gastrostomy, cleaned and reswallowed. The treatments are repeated at intervals of a few days, the olives gradually being increased in size. Quite small children can be induced to swallow the olives, especially if they are smeared with something sweet.

Peptic ulceration of the oesophagus

A peptic ulcer in the oesophagus occurs at its lower end from an upward escape of gastric juice from the stomach. This is common in patients who have a diaphragmatic hernia of the stomach due to a congenital shortening of the oesophagus or to increased abdominal pressure, together with a degeneration of the fibres encircling the oesophagogastric junction.

Symptoms. The symptoms are dysphagia, in addition to those of a gastric ulcer. They are intermittent but progressive. The dysphagia is for solid food. The pain is in the epigastrium and usually penetrates through to the back and often to the left shoulder. Attacks come on shortly after meals or in assuming a recumbent position. Vomiting may bring relief; so will the taking of alkali. Patients usually choose to sleep in the sitting position. Long-continued ulceration will result in narrowing of the oesophagus by scar tissue.

The diagnosis is made by an X-ray study after a barium swallow. Oesophagoscopy is important to show the amount of ulceration and stenosis present, and to exclude carcinoma.

Treatment. The medical treatment is largely dietetic. Stricture is treated by dilatation through an oesophagoscope, or more often, since the disease is progressive, by operation.

Carcinoma of the oesophagus

Cancer of the oesophagus is a comparatively common form of

malignant disease although it seems now to be rarer than it was formerly. It is a most distressing condition, but of recent years surgery of the oesophagus has made great advances, and if the carcinoma can be diagnosed reasonably early, a radical resection of the affected area can be achieved, and in addition, restoration of the alimentary tract is established by means of an oesophagogastric or oesophagojejunal anastomosis or by the use of artificial grafts.

Symptoms. The typical patient is an elderly or middle-aged man, very thin but of good colour, who for some months has suffered from increasing dysphagia. He complains that the food sticks at some point according to the site of the obstruction. The food is often regurgitated after a few minutes. It is undigested, not acid to litmus and has not reached the stomach. The dysphagia is intermittent in carcinoma of the oesophagus and is often ignored by the patient until the taking of solid food is impossible. Pain is usually a late symptom of the disease, so that the malignant condition is rarely discovered early. Therefore, any reported abnormality of swallowing should be investigated by X-rays, the oesophagoscope, and if a lesion is seen, by biopsy and examination of the specimen.

Treatment is carried out in a ward for general surgery and will not be described in detail here. Gastrostomy is best avoided, and if a radical resection is not advisable, radiotherapy can give some temporary relief. Sometimes Souttar's tube, or a similar device made from plastic material, is inserted to enable the patient whose case is hopeless to swallow with relative comfort.

23 Nursing techniques relating to the pharynx, larynx, trachea and oesophagus

Spraying the throat

It is sometimes necessary to spray the throat with a local anaesthetic before a posterior rhinoscopy, endoscopy (especially broncho-scopy), or before dissection of tonsils. The solution used is 10% cocaine, to which may be added 0.06 ml of adrenaline 1 in 1000; 1 ml of the cocaine solution is usually sufficient, and the maximum anaesthetic effect occurs about 15 minutes after application.

Method. The patient is first given a mouthwash. The solution is put into a Roger's spray and the tongue is sprayed. This is then held down whilst the pharynx and epiglottis are sprayed.

An alternative, and more generally used, method of anaesthetiz-ing the throat is to give the patient a tablet of benzocaine or amethocaine to suck 20 minutes before the examination.

After-care. The patient should not be given any food or fluid until the effects of the cocaine have worn off. A mouthwash can be given to freshen the mouth and to remove any unpleasant taste.

Nursing care following endoscopy

Sedation

It is normal to sedate the patient prior to endoscopic examination. The effects of the sedation may cause the patient to be drowsy even up to 24 hours after the examination. The patient should be prevented from injury during this time. Out-patients should be advised not to drive or work with machinery. Alcohol must not be consumed for at least 24 hours, as it enhances the sedation.

Local anaesthesia

As previously mentioned, hot fluids should be avoided for the first 24 hours after local anaesthesia. Great care must be taken when eating and drinking over the first twelve hours, as hot food or liquid could burn the tissues.

Nasogastric feeding

The nasogastric tube or oesophageal tube is passed in theatre at the end of the operation.

The patient is sat upright in bed and a napkin or drape positioned to protect his clothing. The procedure is explained to him, for it is important that he is aware that this provides his meal.

A syringe is placed onto the tube and a little aspirate is withdrawn and placed in a bowl. Blue litmus is drawn through the aspirate to test that it is gastric juice. This indicates the position of the end of the tube.

The feed as prepared by the dietician may be hot or cold, though the temperature of a hot feed must be tested to avoid burning.

A funnel is then attached to the end of the tube, and the feed slowly instilled. This procedure should not be rushed, for, as already mentioned, it provides the patient's meal.

On completion of the procedure, the tube should be flushed through with water, leaving the tube clear. A fresh spigot is placed on the end of the tube and the tubing secured to the patient's face.

VI Specialized Areas of Ear, Nose and Throat Work

24 The Out-Patients' Department

The Out-Patients' Department is a very important part of an Ear, Nose and Throat Unit. Many patients receive treatment here and do not need admission to the ward. Those who are admitted to the ward are first examined in the Out-Patients' Department, and some minor operative procedures are performed there.

The Department should have an ample waiting hall for patients, so that overcrowding is avoided. It should have adequate ventilation and heating, artificial ventilation being installed in some cases. There should be a number of consulting and examination rooms or cubicles, a small theatre, and a 'short-stay' bed area. In addition, an office for secretarial work should be provided.

The examination room

Furniture

The room in which the patient is examined must frequently be darkened by blinds. Therefore a good artificial light is required. A standard lamp of the angled type is used for inspecting the patient, the light being reflected from a head mirror worn by the surgeon. Alternatively, a head lamp may be used. The patient sits in a chair, of which there are several types. A swivel chair may be used. The standard lamp on a movable stand is placed on the left side of the patient's chair. The surgeon, wearing the head mirror on his forehead, sits opposite the patient. At the surgeon's right hand there should be a table, on which the instruments required for various examinations are laid. At the side of the table there should be a bin, with a lid, for soiled-dressing materials. The lid is operated by a foot-lever, and the bag should be detachable for easy sealing and removing. A supply of stationery, including request forms for pathological investigation and X-ray examination, and instructions for home treatments, should be put in a convenient place; also a supply of paper handkerchiefs and of packets of absorbent paper ('Medical Wipes').

Instruments on examination table

On the table, the instruments should be laid out as follows:

1. The surgeon's head mirror, or head lamp.
2. Cotton wool, of the finest absorbent quality.
3. Jobson–Horne ring probes and aural orange sticks (the wool is wound round these, for the purpose of absorbing moisture from cavities).
4. Clean dressing towel, for drying instruments.
5. Receiver for soiled instruments.
6. Spirit lamp and box of matches. (These are for warming mirrors and specula; some surgeons prefer to use boiling water.)
7. Bowl of Hibitane 7% in spirit for disinfecting mirrors which cannot be boiled.

The instruments required for examination:

8. Nasal specula.
9. Aural specula.
10. Tongue depressors.
11. Laryngeal and post-nasal mirrors.
12. Metal probes or orange sticks.
13. Aural forceps.
14. Nasal forceps.
15. Tuning fork.
16. Pharyngotympanic (Eustachian) catheters.
17. Politzer bag.
18. Auscultation tube, the vulcanite end pieces of which, after use, are placed in Hibitane.
19. Siegle's speculum.
20. Rogers or De Vilbiss spray.

Cleaning of instruments. After use, instruments are scrubbed with a brush under running cold water and, in some departments, in Hibitane (chlorhexidine) solution, after which they must be rinsed. If the hospital has a central supply of sterile articles, they are returned to that department. Otherwise, those which are boilable (not mirrors or vulcanite articles) are then boiled for five minutes in water to which bicarbonate of soda may have been added in the proportion of 5 ml to 1 litre of water. Mirrors must never be boiled, unless marked 'boilable'. They may be dipped quickly into boiling water and then immersed in Hibitane 75% in spirit for at least 20 minutes in order to disinfect them and are then rinsed in plain water and dried.

Wooden spatulae and orange sticks are broken after use, and thrown into the bin for soiled dressings.

At the end of the day, all instruments should be dried and carefully examined; those needed repair should be placed on one side and the matter reported to the sister in charge. New nurses should be warned that the angle of a post-nasal mirror is intentional, and that they should not, in their zeal, attempt to straighten it!

Drugs on examination table

1. Cocaine hydrochloride 10% solution.
2. Adrenaline 1 in 1000 solution.
3. Anaesthetic lozenges, e.g. amethocaine.
4. Cocaine paste 25%.
5. Ephedrine 1%.
6. Hydrargaphen (Penotrane) 0.4% in absorbent starch base powder in an insufflator.
7. Antibiotic preparations.
8. Hydrocortisone and neomycin ointment.

Preparing a patient for examination

Ideally, the examiner and all attendants should be masked.

Inspection of the face as a whole may have a bearing upon nasal conditions.

Mouth breathing is revealed by the shape of the mouth, which is narrowed and held open. Blockage of the nasal passage, such as occurs with enlarged adenoids, leads to constant sniffing on the part of the child, and this causes suction on the roof of the mouth which results in arching of the palate, a narrow jaw, and overlapping of the incisor teeth. The facial appearance is generally termed 'adenoid facies' (Fig. 24.1).

Collapse or expansion of the alae nasi, widening of the bridge of the nose, fulness over the accessory sinuses, or soreness of the vestibule and upper lip, are frequent indications of nasal infection.

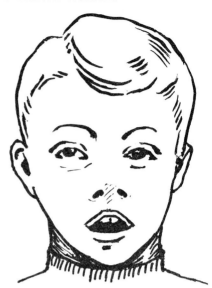

Fig. 24.1. *The adenoid facies.*

When a child is to be examined, a few minutes spent in gaining his or her confidence may often avoid struggles. If the nurse is required to hold the child, she should realize that she can neither gain his co-operation nor restrain his head movements by grasping his hands. The correct method of holding him is to wrap a towel or blanket round him to restrain his arm and hand movements. He is then sat on her knee, facing the medical practitioner. The nurse can steady the child's head with one hand, and use her shoulder to support the back of his head and neck (see Fig. 24.2). An adult's head is usually steadied between the hands of the nurse, who stands behind him.

Examination of the nose

It is usually the nurse's duty to dress the probes immediately before they are required. If prepared long in advance, the wool may become loose. Cotton wool of a long-fibred absorbent quality is used. It is especially teased for the purpose, and may be provided in sterilized cartons. If a wooden carrier is moistened first, the wool will adhere more firmly. A wisp is placed on the end of the probe so that part projects in a loose tuft; the remainder is twisted firmly round the probe. The nurse should test it to ensure that the wool will not become dislodged during use.

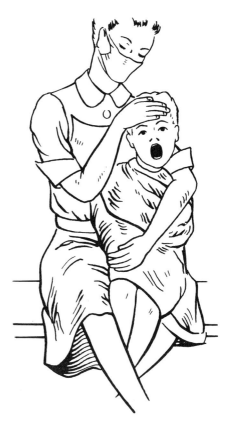

Fig. 24.2. *Holding a child for a throat examination.*

Taking a swab of the anterior nares

No treatment should be applied to the area for at least six hours beforehand.

The patient is seated facing a good light. A sterile swab is taken from a sterile test tube, passed into one nostril for 25–50 mm and rubbed gently but firmly round the nasal fossa. If a membrane is present the swab should be placed on it. The swab is then withdrawn and replaced in the sterile tube, which must be suitably labelled and sent to the laboratory without delay.

Sometimes swabs may be required from both nostrils, in which case they should be marked 'Left' and 'Right'.

Taking a post-nasal swab

This procedure may be carried out on persons suspected of carrying the meningococcus of cerebrospinal meningitis. The oral route is used, and a swab mounted on a bent wire is employed.

A good light is essential. The tongue should be depressed by a spatula, so that the swab can be directed to the required position without touching the sensitive uvula and without becoming contaminated with saliva (see Fig. 24.3).

Bacteria commonly found in the nose and throat include *Streptococcus viridans*, *Neisseria catarrhalis*, and various micrococci.

Infective organisms include haemolytic streptococci, pneumococci, influenzal bacilli, *corynebacterium diphtheriae*, staphylococci and viruses. *Candida albicans*, which causes thrush, may follow the use of broad-spectrum antibiotics.

Aural discharge in acute otitis media may contain influenzal

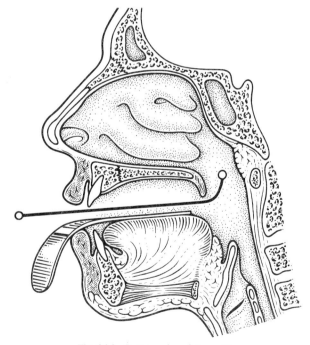

Fig. 24.3. *Post-nasal swab in position.*

bacilli, pneumococci or other streptococci, and staphylococci; in chronic otitis media it frequently contains staphylococci, *Bacillus proteus*, and *Pseudomonas pyocyanea*. Occasionally, there are certain species of fungus — notably the aspergillus species.

For some examinations, the nose may require spraying or preliminary packing in order to anaesthetize it.

Before examination of the ear, the outer ear may need syringing to clear it of wax. These nursing techniques are also carried out in the ward, and are described in the appropriate chapters.

Examination of the ear

The external aspect of the ear gives little or no information as to its internal condition. Radiography may show this to a certain extent. A mastoid abscess may cause bulging behind the auricle and push it forward.

To test hearing, tuning forks of varying pitch are required. These help to indicate degrees of deafness and whether the cause lies in the middle or the inner ear.

Examination of the tympanum

The normal eardrum is a grey transparent membrane closing the inner end of the external auditory canal and lying at an angle with it in a double slant. It is a tense membrane (hence the name 'drum'). Through the eardrum can be seen the malleus of the middle ear and below this a cone of light (reflected light) spreads downwards. After syringing the ear, the healthy eardrum often appears pink. With infection it becomes first red and later opaque and thickened. Swelling of the meatus may obstruct the view of the eardrum.

Before examination, the ear should be inspected (Fig. 24.4). Any wax, pus or debris should be removed and the meatus dried. Syringing is the best method, but must be used only on the instruction of a doctor. The procedure is carried out by nursing staff who have written authorization from their employing authority.

Examination with head mirror and speculum

The patient should be sitting if possible. Several sizes of speculum should be available. The examiner holds the warmed speculum

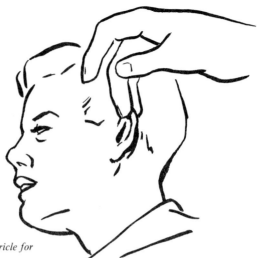

Fig. 24.4. *Holding the auricle for
examination of the ear.*

between his thumb and forefinger and inserts it into the meatus,
which is straightened by drawing the auricle up and back with the
middle and ring fingers. For an infant, the auricle is drawn down and
back, as the bone is not fully developed. The nurse shines a light into
the head mirror. A mirror is unnecessary with an electric auriscope,
which also gives a magnified image.

In some ear diseases the eardrum is indrawn or bound by
adhesions. To test its mobility, *Siegle's speculum* is used. This
instrument consists of a rubber bulb and tube, to which is attached
an end-piece into which is screwed a lens. This lens is warmed over a
spirit lamp, to prevent condensation of moisture upon it.

An aural speculum is fitted to the end-piece and inserted into the
ear. If the bulb is compressed when inserting the speculum,
relaxation of the bulb, by producing a negative pressure in the
meatus, will tend to draw the eardrum outwards. By varying the air
pressure, an otherwise invisible perforation may be detected.

The condition of the pharyngotympanic (Eustachian) tube, which
may be obstructed or may contain mucus, is investigated by inflation
of the middle ear.

1. Valsalva's method. The patient should close his mouth, nip his nostrils and try to blow forcibly. If the tubes are patent, air is forced up them and he will hear a click as air enters the middle ear. The examiner may confirm this by watching through a speculum for movement of the tympanum, or listening via an auscultation tube.

2. Politzer's method. This method is used most often on children. The child holds a sip of water in his mouth. The nozzle of the Politzer's bag is inserted into one nostril and then both are closed so that no air can escape. The child is told to swallow and at the moment of swallowing, the bag is compressed and air is driven into the middle ear. During swallowing the orifices of the pharyngotympanic tubes are opened; the soft palate rises and shuts off the nasopharynx from the parts below.

3. Inflation by pharyngotympanic catheter. In this method one tube only is inflated at a time. The metal catheter, usually silver, has a curved beak to fit into the orifice of the pharyngotympanic tube, and at the other end, a ring on the same side as the curve, to indicate its position when hidden. The catheter is passed along the floor of the nose until it touches the posterior pharyngeal wall. It is then turned point outwards and gently withdrawn until it passes into the pharyngotympanic tube. An air bag is then attached to the catheter, and air driven gently up the tube. An auscultation tube may be attached to a stethoscope connecting the ear of the patient with that of the surgeon who can then hear the air blowing into the middle ear if the pharyngotympanic tube is patent. Bubbling sounds indicate the presence of pus; a whistling sound, a perforation of the drum.

The auscultation tube is fitted at each end with a vulcanite end-piece — one black and one white. The surgeon usually chooses the white end-piece to place in his own ear.

The nurse should be very careful over the cleaning and drying of the catheters. Being made of soft metal, they bend easily and may become dented with rough handling. After cleaning, air should be blown through with the Politzer bag to make sure that they are patent.

Before examining the ear of a very young child, a general anaesthetic is given; a pharyngotympanic catheter is passed via the nose by the surgeon, and the tube is inflated whilst the surgeon examines the ear with an auriscope.

Examination of the throat

The larynx cannot normally be seen by direct vision; however, by passing an illuminated tube-spatula, the soft tissues of the throat can be so displaced that the interior of the larynx and its surrounding parts can be seen. This is called 'direct laryngoscopy'. 'Indirect laryngoscopy' is the examination by means of a mirror and will be described here. The patient may be recumbent or sitting, with his head extended. The method of holding a child has already been described. The nurse stands or sits behind the patient so that he does not back away from the surgeon. A good light is essential and a hand lamp or torch may be needed.

If examining with a torch only, a tongue depressor should be placed over the centre of the tongue, pushing it gently down. It should not be placed far back, as this may make the patient retch. If a laryngeal mirror is used, the tongue is held forward in a paper tissue. The mirror is warmed in the water or in the flame of the spirit lamp. This prevents 'misting' by the patient's breath.

The examiner should test the heat of the mirror on his own hand or cheek before putting it in the patient's mouth. During the examination, he asks the patient to say 'ee-ee', as this causes approximation of the vocal cords.

25 Radiotherapy

Radiotherapy is the treatment of disease with X-rays or gamma rays. These have a selective action on malignant cells and cause damage to the nucleus, preventing cell division. There is also some temporary damage to normal cells which shows itself as the radiation reaction, but if the dose of X-rays is carefully regulated, this reaction settles down quickly and a cure results.

It is important to keep the irradiated area small in order to produce as little disturbance to the patient as possible. In the tongue, this can be done by implanting radioactive needles or seeds directly into the tumour. If, however, the growth has spread more extensively or has involved the glands of the neck, it is preferable to use X-rays administered externally.

For many years radium was the only radioactive material available and when first produced it was extremely expensive and was guarded with care by the nursing staff. After the invention of the atom bomb, nuclear reactors were developed and materials such as radioactive gold, iridium, cobalt, caesium, strontium and yttrium became available. These can be produced in larger quantities, and are used as alternatives to radium. The rays they produce are not so penetrating and simplify storage and protection problems.

It is important for the nurse to realize what dangers are associated with radioactivity, but at the same time to keep these in perspective. The more actively dividing tissues are most sensitive to radiation and large doses can affect the blood and ovaries, causing anaemia and sterility. These doses are never likely to be reached with the small amount of radium used in needle implantation treatments and even the patient will not be affected in this way.

Staff who are responsible for the safety of radioactive materials are specially designated and have routine checks of radiation received. This ensures that they do not receive more than the tolerance dose which is laid down by the authorities. The nurse who looks after the occasional case is not likely to reach this dose and is not usually tested in this way.

Implantation techniques

Radium

In this method needles containing radium are inserted in a planned pattern to produce uniform dosage throughout the tumour. The needles are made of platinoiridium and contain from 0.5 to 3 mg of radium inside an inner platinum cell. They are threaded on silk to enable them to be removed.

A general anaesthetic is given and the position of the needles checked by an X-ray. The needles are left in place for a week and are examined twice a day to ensure that none is working loose. The threads are usually secured firmly to the cheek by strapping and should not be disturbed.

A chart showing the number and type of needles is kept in the notes and a special sign showing the presence of radioactivity is displayed at the foot of the bed. During this time visitors may be allowed, but they should not sit close to the bed and should be discouraged from lengthy visits.

The nursing treatment whilst the needles are in place is chiefly directed towards maintaining the patient's nutrition and keeping the mouth as clean as possible. A special liquid diet can be provided, but it is often more convenient and certainly more palatable to put the normal diet through a liquidizer, to break down solid particles. After each meal the mouth should be irrigated with normal saline, to wash food particles away from the needles and their threads.

At the end of the calculated time the needles are removed, usually by the medical staff, and returned to the safe. If they are placed far back in the tongue, an anaesthetic may be required. They are carefully counted, and as an extra precaution the patient is surveyed with a portable radiation monitor to be quite sure that all radium has been removed.

Radioactive gold

This has a short half-life of 2.8 days and therefore becomes largely inactive after 2 to 3 weeks. It is used in the form of small 'seeds', 3 mm long, which can be implanted into the tissues and left there permanently. These seeds are put in with a special gun carrying a cartridge of 15 seeds. They do not interfere with movements of the tongue and little special nursing care is required. The patient needs only a short stay in hospital, usually two or three days.

Radioactive iridium

In this technique, nylon tubes are inserted into the tongue and their position checked by an X-ray before they are loaded with the radioactive iridium wire. This cuts down the exposure to medical and nursing staff in the Theatre and X-ray departments.

X-ray therapy

When the tumour is no longer localized to a small area, external X-ray therapy is used. There is no difference in the action of the gamma rays from radium and the X-rays produced by electrical machines. It is merely a question of how deep into the tissues they penetrate, and this depends on the voltage at which the X-rays are generated.

Deep X-rays produced at 250 000 volts have been used for many years, but they are now being replaced by X-rays from linear accelerators at 4–6 million volts or by the rays from radioactive cobalt. Both these have the advantage that they cause little skin reaction and can easily penetrate bone and cartilage which may be involved with tumour. The less penetrating deep X-rays tended to be absorbed by these tissues which were therefore overdosed, causing pain and necrosis. The development of new equipment for radiotherapy has greatly reduced the discomfort of X-ray therapy.

It is still necessary to treat as small an area as possible and often a special jig or mask is constructed for each individual patient, so that several beams of X-rays can be accurately directed to the tumour site. Treatment is given over four to five weeks, often on an outpatient basis, and the daily progress of tumour and reaction are observed.

An optimistic and encouraging attitude is essential during this extended treatment, especially when the inevitable discomfort of the reaction begins. Radiation to the mouth and neck reduces the amount of saliva and mucus and causes a dry mouth and loss of taste.

Two-hourly fluid or soft feeds should be advised and the patient should also be encouraged to drink as much as possible of bland fluids. He will not want to eat very hot or seasoned foods. Moreover, 14 g of mucilage containing 500 mg of aspirin given half an hour before meals makes swallowing very much easier.

The skin reaction is not usually a problem, but the soreness and redness of the erythema can be reduced by a spray containing hydrocortisone. Skin marks used in the planning of the treatment should not be washed off without medical permission. When large areas of the trunk or abdomen are treated the patient may have a general reaction, with headache and nausea. This is not a problem where only the neck area is treated. If the patient feels sick or nauseated in any way he should be treated with chlorpromazine hydrochloride (Largactil) or perphenazine (Fentazin).

Hyperbaric oxygen therapy

It is now known that large tumour masses have areas that are poorly supplied with blood vessels, where the cells are lacking in oxygen. This makes them difficult to kill with radiation and the centre of the tumour may require a higher dose than the normal tissues can stand.

The problem is to get more oxygen to the blood stream and from this to the anoxic cells. This can be achieved by increasing the pressure at which oxygen is breathed. A special hyperbaric chamber of perspex, in which the patient lies during treatment, is used. He wears special antistatic clothing, to minimize the risk of sparking and subsequent fire. The pressure is increased gradually over the first 15 minutes until 3 atmospheres is reached and this is maintained for a further 15 minutes to allow oxygen to soak through the tissues. Treatment is then given through the wall. During the whole of this time the radiographer talks to the patient through the headphones. As the pressure increases the patient is told to swallow to prevent pressure changes in the ears. Some radiotherapists perform a myringotomy before treatment and insert grommets into the eardrums to avoid pressure changes and subsequent pain. This, however, is not essential.

The oxygen method is still under trial in many centres and is not universally available. Initial results suggest that it may be very useful in tumours around the head and neck.

Further reading

Ballantyne J.C. (1978) *A Synopsis of Otolaryngology*, 3rd edn. Bristol: J. Wright.
Beagley H.A. (1982) *Manual of Audiometric Techniques*. Oxford: Oxford University Press.
Birrell J.F. (ed.) (1977) *Logan Turner's Diseases of the Nose, Throat and Ear*, 8th edn. Bristol: J. Wright.
Bull T.P. (1978) *Recent Advances in Otolaryngology*. Edinburgh: Churchill Livingstone.
Foxen E.H.M. (1980) *Lecture Notes on Diseases of the Ear, Nose and Throat*, 5th edn. Oxford: Blackwell Scientific Publications.
Hall I.S. and Colman B.H. (1981) *Diseases of the Nose, Throat and Ear*, 12th edn. Edinburgh: Churchill Livingstone.
Smyth G.D.L. (1980) *Chronic Ear Disease*, Vol. 2. Edinburgh: Churchill Livingstone.

Appendix A
Some important drugs used in ear, nose and throat nursing

Local anaesthetics

Local anaesthetics may be used to produce complete insensibility to pain in a particular area of the body. One of the drugs most frequently used for this purpose is *cocaine*. Cocaine has little action on the unbroken skin, but if applied to mucous membrane it produces complete local anaesthesia, so that small operations can be performed without the patients feeling them. For ear, nose and throat work the drug is commonly used in strengths of 10–25% aqueous solution of cocaine hydrochloride. Not only does its power of penetrating mucous surfaces make it an efficient anaesthetic, but the vasoconstriction that it induces is of great value, particularly in the nose. The consequent shrinkage of the mucous membrane improves visibility and access to the passages and assists sinus drainage. The action of the drug is increased and prolonged by the addition of 0.06 ml of adrenaline solution 1 in 1000 to each 1.3 ml of cocaine used.

In place of the cocaine solution, which is sprayed on mucous surfaces, cocaine paste is frequently used. This is a compound of cocaine (usually 25%) and suprarenal extract in a mixture of liquid paraffin and petroleum jelly. The great advantages of this paste are that it keeps indefinitely and that the absorption of cocaine is minimal.

Owing to its toxicity and its tendency to produce addiction cocaine is listed as a Controlled Drug and can be obtained only on the signed prescription of a doctor. It must be kept in a locked cupboard, within a locked cupboard, which is used only for Controlled Drugs.

The toxic effects are pallor, sweating, shallow breathing and a fall in blood pressure. The pulse at first quickens, then becomes slow and feeble. There may be nausea and vomiting, and should cerebral irritation occur there are convulsions. Death may follow from heart failure or from asphyxia. Cocaine is especially dangerous to children under six years of age, and for all ages it is too toxic for injection into the tissues. The first-aid treatment for cocaine reaction is to lower the patient's head, loosen the clothing round his neck, open a nearby window and give oxygen. If the patient can swallow, he may be given water, sal volatile or brandy. The most up-to-date remedy is intravenous thiopentone sodium.

For local anaesthesia produced by subcutaneous injection cocaine has been largely superseded by substitutes such as procaine and amethocaine. These are less effective as surface anaesthetics but are less toxic and do not produce addiction. They are not subject to Controlled Drug Regulations, but the dose must be adequately checked at the time of administration. A so-called idiosyncrasy to a local anaesthetic is probably due to accidental absorption into the blood stream either during injection or through a wound in the mucous membrane to which the anaesthetic is applied. To avoid the possibility of cerebral disturbances, all patients due to have a local anaesthetic of cocaine should be given a barbiturate, such as 100 mg of pentobarbitone sodium (Nembutal) the night before. The adrenaline that some surgeons add to the cocaine solution is used in order to diminish local absorption of cocaine.

Cocaine may cause excitement in some patients, and if used in the treatment of an out-patient, he should be allowed to rest for at least half an hour before leaving hospital.

After the throat has been cocainized for direct endoscopy, the cough reflex will be absent for some time, and special precautions must be taken that the patient does not inhale fluid or food. Nothing is given by mouth for two hours, then the patient is given a glass of water to sip slowly.

Drugs to combat infection

The discovery this century of drugs that will harm invading organisms more than living tissue has revolutionized the treatment of infection. The two main groups of these drugs — sulphonamides and antibiotics — are bacteriostatic or bacteriodical according to their concentration. Sulphonamides act by competing for the raw materials necessary for the existence of the organisms. The result is that, since the bacteria are prevented from growing and multiplying, the natural defences of the body can deal with them. When the influence of the drug is withdrawn, the remaining organisms resume growth and multiplication. The aim is to keep the drug in contact with the infected tissue until the infection is overcome. Antibiotics act more directly. Some will block an essential enzyme, but penicillin, for instance, acts on the cell wall of the bacterium, causing it to rupture under osmotic pressure. Others act directly on bacterial cell contents. The drugs are rapidly absorbed and eliminated (although there are newer longer-acting compounds) or diffuse rapidly from any site of local application; therefore repeated administration during this period is necessary.

The essential value of these drugs is in the treatment of acute infection. They are relatively ineffective in chronic infections, more particularly in chronic types of disease, possibly because these are often of an allergic rather than an infective nature. In all cases, resistant strains of organisms occur, and laboratory tests must be made to discover the agents to which the organisms are sensitive.

Chemotherapy — Sulphonamides

Systemic treatment by a sulpha drug may be used as an alternative to an antibiotic for serious streptococcal infections particularly where there is danger of meningitis, but its use is uncommon for pharyngitis of average severity, since in the first place, neither the duration nor the severity of the disease is markedly lessened by its use, and, in the second, the possible dangers inherent in the use of these drugs are greater than those of the infection. If sulpha therapy is considered advisable, the preparations usually chosen are *sulphadiazine* or *sulphadimidine* (Sulphamezathine), the latter being the less toxic. Both are rapidly absorbed and eliminated, therefore large initial doses are ordered, followed by smaller maintenance doses which must be given both night and day. A usual prescription is 2–4 g to be given at once, then 1.5 g 4-hourly until symptoms subside. A sodium bicarbonate mixture is frequently ordered with each dose. For children, the amount of sulpha is calculated by their weight, giving 0.2 g per kg per day. The amount of the drug given must be recorded. Sulphonamides (usually sulphadiazine) are the treatment of choice in meningitis because of the ease with which they cross into the cerebrospinal fluid.

During the prolonged administration of a sulpha drug a large amount of fluid should be taken by the patient in order to prevent crystallization in the kidneys. (This complication, however, is extremely rare with sulphamezathine.) The amount of fluid intake and output should be recorded, and the urine tested daily. Should haematuria or anuria occur, the drug must be stopped at once, but the alkaline mixture should be continued. The doctor must be informed immediately.

Another rare danger of sulpha therapy is agranulocytosis. Nearly every patient gets some reduction of leucocytes, which usually appears after six days. Should an early reduction occur, the drug is discontinued. The same applies if fever has not abated after 48 hours.

Sulpha drugs may produce toxic effects in a person sensitized by previous administration, which is another argument against the routine use of the drugs in mild infections. These toxic effects include high fever, cyanosis, skin rashes, a red sore throat, headache, loss of appetite, nausea and vomiting.

Antibiotics

These are drugs prepared from living moulds or other bacteria, and constitute the most recent group of drugs to be used against infection. Their action depends on the inhibitory effect exerted by one organism on another — 'antibiosis'. During the past few years, many such drugs have been used because of their activity against different organisms. The most important of these are:

Penicillin, effective against Gram-positive organisms and certain spirochaetes.

Streptomycin, effective against Gram-negative organisms and certain acid-fast bacilli.

Ampicillin
  (Penbritin)
Chloramphenicol
  (Chloromycetin)
Tetracycline
  (Achromycin)
Oxytetracycline
  (Terramycin)
Chlortetracycline
  (Aureomycin)

These are called 'broad-spectrum' antibiotics, being effective against many organisms, including some large viruses. Since they tend to sterilize the small intestine, large doses of vitamin B are usually given if the drugs are used over a prolonged period.

Erythromycin
Neomycin
Nystatin   This antibiotic is specific for fungal
                             organisms.

Methicillin Sodium   ⎫
  (Celbenin)   ⎬ Used for resistant staphylococci.
Cloxacillin Sodium   ⎭
  (Orbenin)

Penicillin is frequently used, partly because it is cheap, and partly because, apart from the hypersensitivity which some people develop towards it, it is relatively non-toxic. It is given by deep intramuscular injection. One scheme is to give a high dose of crystalline pencillin, for example 500 000 units or even 1–2 000 000 units, followed by a similar dose 12 hours later. The theory is that the first dose produces a high level in the blood and is excreted in four hours, and the second dose produces another high level, when any remaining organisms are ready to divide. This method removes the need for frequent needle-pricks. Other methods involve the six- or eight-hourly doses of 300 000 to 1 000 000 units of one of the more slowly absorbed preparations over several days. Capsules and tablets for oral use are widely prescribed. Should several courses of these tablets be required, then vitamin B may also be prescribed. This is needed because non-pathogenic bacteria normally living in the colon and helping in the absorption of vitamin B are destroyed by oral antibiotics.

Penicillin must be kept cold when in solution, although the crystals in a dry state are fairly stable. In the presence of water the drug rapidly loses its effect and contamination with organisms from the hand can destroy its effect. Therefore, the nurse should use a disposable sterile syringe and an aseptic procedure for preparing and giving the injection. At the same time, in order to avoid developing hypersensitivity to the drug, she should keep all traces of penicillin solution off her own hands. Any excess solution drawn into the syringe should be returned to the phial before withdrawing the needle — it should not be squirted into the air.

Streptomycin. This antibiotic may be used to combat certain organisms that are insensitive to penicillin, notably the tubercle bacillus. It has not been used to a great extent in ear, nose and throat work except for tuberculous conditions. Streptomycin has an effect on both the vestibular and auditory functions of the inner ear, and deafness has several times been attributed to its use. The usual dosage of streptomycin is 0.5 g twice daily until 15 g has been given. The drug is then discontinued except in tuberculosis.

Chlortetracycline (Aureomycin). This drug differs from the preceding antibiotics in that it is usually given by mouth. It is particularly useful against *Staphylococcus aureus*. Although it is not absorbed so quickly into the blood as is penicillin, it disappears more slowly. The usual dosage is 0.5–1 g every four hours until 12–14 g have been given.

Chloramphenicol (Chloromycetin). This drug was originally derived from a mould, but is now prepared synthetically. Like chlortetracycline, it is given by mouth, usually in capsular form, though it can be absorbed rectally. Unlike chlortetracycline, it contains a nitrobenzine factor in its composition, which can cause a severe form of anaemia, and therefore it should be prescribed with caution. It is recommended that its use should be reserved for the diseases for which it is specifically valuable—whooping cough and infections shown to be sensitive to it in laboratory tests.

Oxytetracycline (Terramycin). This is still another antibiotic, useful when organisms are penicillin-resistant. It can be given by mouth— 2 g daily for fourteen days, and is also prepared as a 1% ointment or in powder form for insufflation.

Neomycin. This is an antibiotic too toxic to be given by mouth or injection, but useful as a local application in ears because it acts on *Pseudomonas pyocyanea*. It is an ointment, often combined with cortisone.

Orbenin and **Celbenin** are given by injection.

Polymyxin. This is the name given to a group of five polypeptide antibiotics produced from *Bacillus polymyxa* and named A to E. Polymyxin B is the best of the series and is effective against many organisms including *Pseudomonas pyocyanea* and *Escherichia coli*. It is used for local or general treatment and prepared as 1% drops, 2%

ointment or for parenteral injection. The usual course is 250 000 units intramuscularly every four hours for five days.

For severe infections of the ear, nose or throat, it is customary to prescribe an antibiotic immediately. At the same time, laboratory tests are made to discover whether the organisms responsible for the infection are sensitive or resistant to the drugs used. Guidance can then be given as to the type of drug and the dosage which would be most helpful.

There is need for co-operation between the ward and laboratory to control hospital infection. Genetic changes in bacteria can cause significant alterations in the infection pattern.

Cytotoxic agents

Certain malignant conditions of the head and neck may be treated by drugs known as cytotoxic agents. These drugs interfere with the cell metabolism, and malignant cells are particularly sensitive to their effects. Considerable destruction and regression of tumour tissue has been achieved by their use. They are highly toxic and dosage should be carefully controlled. Frequent blood counts are needed as a leucocytosis will occur. Nurses should be aware of the side-effects and should watch for and report these. Side-effects include skin rashes, urticaria, nausea, vomiting and diarrhoea. Severe gingivitis is sometimes seen. Frequent mouth care is necessary for the patient's comfort.

Methotrexate

This is an antimetabolite. Absorption is rapid and the drug is excreted unchanged within 12 hours. Oral tablets of 2.5 mg are used. For parenteral use sodium methotrexate is prepared in 5 and 50 mg vials; it must be reconstituted with water. In treating tumours of the tongue and glands of neck it can be given by continuous intra-arterial infusion. This method ensures that the tumour receives the maximum dose of the drug. Depending on the site of the tumour, a small-bore cannula can be inserted into the external carotid artery, the superior thyroid or lingual arteries. Fluorescein or methylene blue may be injected to ascertain that the cannula is in the correct position. A dose of 50 mg in 24 hours is usually aimed at. In the whole course about 750 mg are given. A specially adapted infusion apparatus is required to allow the reservoir to be at least 3 m above the patient, to overcome the arterial pressure. Sufficient tubing should be used to allow the patient freedom of movement, as the infusion may continue many days. Toxic effects may be lessened by giving folic acid systemically.

Mustines

Nitrogen mustard can be given by simple arterial injection. Phenylalanine may be used also. As soon as the leucocyte count returns to normal, oral therapy may be substituted.

Appendix B
Glossary of instruments

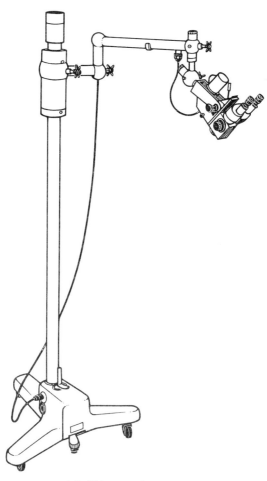

A.1. *Zeiss operating microscope.*

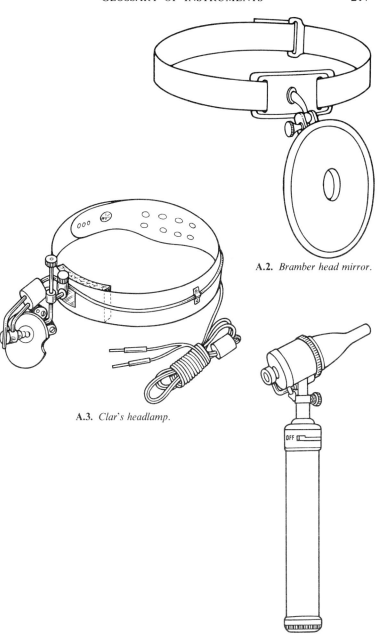

A.2. *Bramber head mirror.*

A.3. *Clar's headlamp.*

A.4. *Auriscope.*

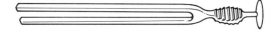
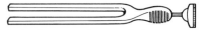

A.5. *Gardiner Brown's tuning fork.*

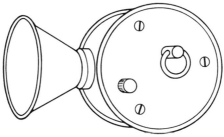

A.6. *Barany's noise box.*

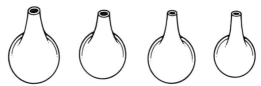

A.7. *Gruber's aural speculum.*

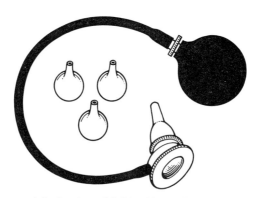

A.8. *Peter's modified Siegle's aural speculum.*

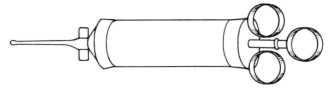

A.9. *Aural syringe.*

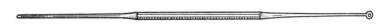

A.10. *Jobson Horne's probe.*

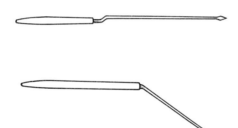

A.11. *Fagge's myringotome and Politzer's myringotome.*

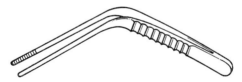

A.12. *Wilde's aural forceps.*

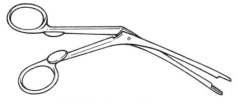

A.13. *Heath's aural forceps.*

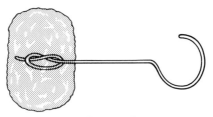

A.14. *Schuknecht gelfoam wire.*

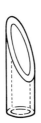

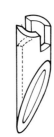

A.15. *Shea's stapes replacement strut, polyethylene.*

A.16. *Shea's tricus grip strut, Teflon.*

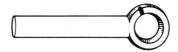

A.17. *Shea's Teflon piston.*

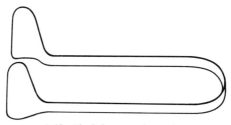

A.18. *Thudichum nasal speculum.*

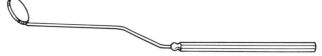

A.19. *St Clair Thomson's nasal mirror.*

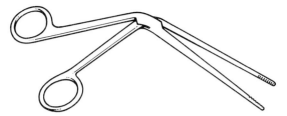

A.20. *Tilley's nasal dressing forceps.*

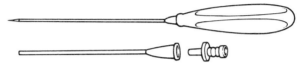

A.21. *Lichtwitz's antrum trocar.*

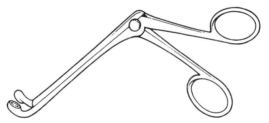

A.22. *Grunwald's nasal punch forceps.*

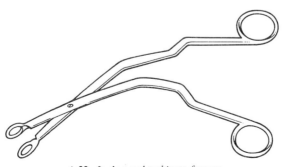

A.23. *Luc's nasal turbinate forceps.*

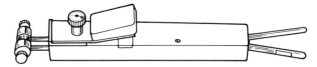

A.24. *Hovell's cautery handle.*

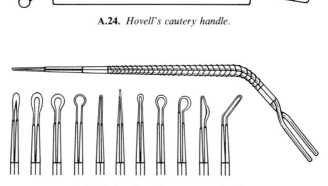

A.25. *Points for galvano-cautery handle.*

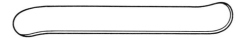

A.26. *Tongue depressor.*

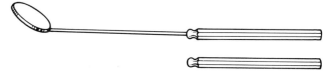

A.27. *Laryngeal mirror.*

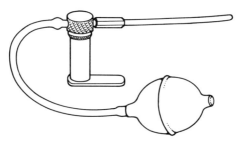

A.28. *Cade's insufflator.*

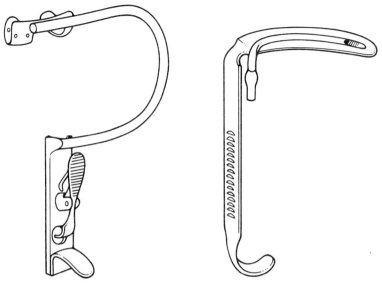

A.29. *Boyle–Davis gag frame.*　　　　　**A.30.** *Boyle–Davis tongue plate.*

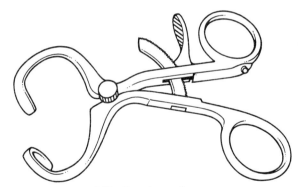

A.31. *Doyen's mouth gag.*

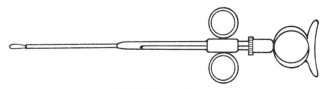

A.32. *Eve's tonsil snare.*

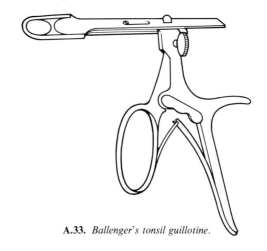

A.33. *Ballenger's tonsil guillotine.*

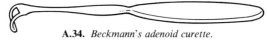

A.34. *Beckmann's adenoid curette.*

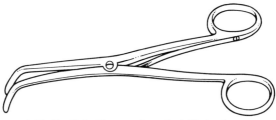

A.35. *Bowlby's (Trousseau) tracheal dilating forceps.*

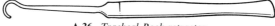
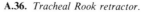

A.36. *Tracheal Rook retractor.*

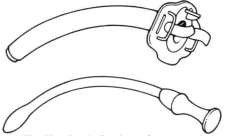

A.37. *Chevalier Jackson's tracheostomy tube.*

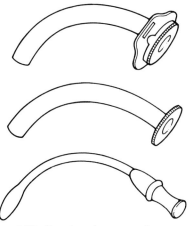

A.38. *Negus' tracheostomy tube.*

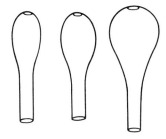

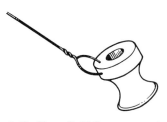

A.39. *Haney & Negus' plastic bobbins.*

A.40. *Shepard's Teflon grommet drain tube.*

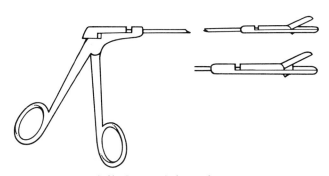

A.41. *Patterson's biopsy forceps.*

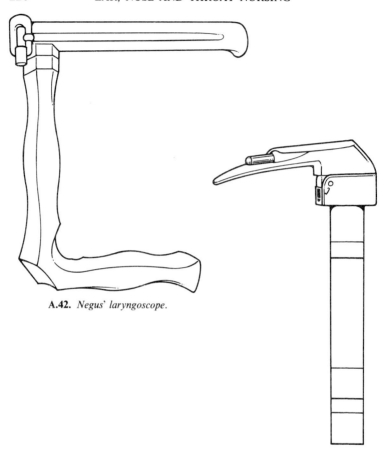

A.42. *Negus' laryngoscope.*

A.43. *Whipps Cross Hospital pattern laryngoscope.*

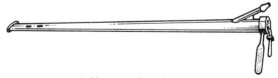

A.44. *Negus' bronchoscope.*

Index